Naturally

A FIRESIDE BOOK
Published by Simon & Schuster
New York London Toronto Sydney

Thin

Unleash Your SkinnyGirl and Free Yourself from a Lifetime of Dieting

Bethenny Frankel

with Eve Adamson

Fireside
A Division of Simon & Schuster, Inc.
1230 Avenue of the Americas
New York, NY 10020

First Fireside trade paperback edition March 2009

FIRESIDE and colophon are registered trademarks of Simon & Schuster, Inc.

For information about special discounts for bulk purchases,
please contact Simon & Schuster Special Sales at 1-800-456-6798
or business@simonandschuster.com

Designed by Nicola Ferguson

Manufactured in the United States of America

10   9   8   7   6   5   4   3   2

Library of Congress Cataloging-in-Publication Data

Frankel, Bethenny.
    Naturally thin : unleash your skinnygirl and free yourself from a lifetime of dieting / Bethenny Frankel with Eve Adamson.
        p.   cm.
    "A Fireside Book."
    1. Weight loss.   2. Nutrition.   3. Food habits.   I. Adamson, Eve.   II. Title.
    RM222.2.F695   2009
    613.2'5—dc22   2008042790

ISBN-13: 978-1-4165-9798-8
ISBN-10:   1-4165-9798-0

This book is dedicated to every girl who wants to be naturally thin but can't stand the thought of dieting even one more day, of starting tomorrow, of obsessing, of feeling guilty or being "good" or "bad." This book is for every girl who fears skinny jeans or a bikini or looking amazing or being the best girl she can be. Every one of you is a skinnygirl dying to break out. If you want it, go get it. I know that you will because you deserve it. You go girl!

Contents

CONTENTS

Introduction

WHO I AM AND WHAT THIS BOOK IS ALL ABOUT

"I look fat. I hate my body." "My thighs are huge." "Why did I just eat that? I can't believe I just ate that." "I can't lose weight. I have a slow metabolism." "I can't eat that. I really want to eat that, but I shouldn't." "I hate myself." "I pigged out." "I'm definitely going on a diet tomorrow." "I can't stay on a diet. I'm hopeless." "I have no will-power. I'm pathetic." "What is wrong with me?" "She can eat anything she wants. I hate her." "I was so good today. I skipped dinner. I can't wait to weigh myself tomorrow and see how much weight I lost." "Tomorrow I'm not eating anything." "I'm never eating again." "I'm not going to that party. I'll just eat too much." "Why did I eat so much? I want a do-over. I feel so guilty." "I can just feel myself getting fatter right now. I'm disgusting." "I would be happy if I could just get skinny."

Sound familiar?

These are not the words or thoughts of a naturally thin person, but they might be the words or thoughts you say to yourself. I used to talk to myself like this, but I don't do it anymore. Do you wish you could stop, too?

You can stop. You can stop it all: the negative talk, the hatred of yourself and your body, the fear of food, the obsession with food, and, most important, the *dieting*. Best of all, when you stop doing all these things to yourself, you will become naturally thin.

If you are so used to thinking about yourself and about food in this negative way, if you feel shackled to diets and you think that this will never change, take heart. Life doesn't have to be this way. You are about to break the vicious circle and escape from a lifetime of self-destructive dieting. You can break free from the oppression of food obsession. And you can become naturally thin, without ever dieting again. I did it, and you can do it, too.

You Are Naturally Thin

Here's the simple truth: millions of Americans have become enslaved by dieting. We torture ourselves constantly, just because we ate a cookie (or five cookies), or didn't go to the gym, or ordered french fries, or had a second helping, or ate carbs or sugar or meat, or can't fit into our skinny jeans, or aren't as skinny as the next person. We insult ourselves and hate ourselves because we don't look the way we think we are supposed to look. We don't feel good or happy or satisfied with our lives, and we blame it all on a number on the scale. We spend thousands of dollars on diet programs, food delivery services, diet Web sites, diet magazines, and diet books. And yet we keep getting fatter. We despair, we wonder what is wrong with us, but we keep on dieting, we keep on trying, and we keep on failing.

If you wish desperately that you were one of those *naturally thin* people, but you don't really believe, deep down, that you are, guess what.

It's all a misconception. Being naturally thin isn't some state of being beyond your grasp. *You are naturally thin*. You just have to make a few simple changes to let your natural thinness emerge. *You* will be one of those people you wished you could be in high school. *You* will be one of those people that others look at and wonder, "How does she stay so thin?" This book will grant you access to that world because deep down, I know that's who you are. I found the secrets, I got *naturally thin* for life, and I want to share those secrets with you.

Who am I? Why am I writing this book? And, perhaps most important, why should you listen to anything *I* have to say about what *you* should eat?

My name is Bethenny Frankel. By trade, I'm a natural foods chef. You might know me from my role on Bravo's *The Real Housewives of New York City*, or from my appearance as a contestant on *Martha Stewart: Apprentice*. You might have read one of my health blogs, seen one of my YouTube videos about healthy cooking, or read my column in *Health* magazine. Maybe you've even tasted some of my healthy treats in my line of baked goods, BethennyBakes™. But what you don't know about me is what I want to share with you: why I'm naturally thin, and why so many of the celebrity clients I cook for are naturally thin, too.

It's no state secret, but somehow, the key to being naturally thin has eluded many American women. I want to change all that. *Everybody* should be able to know and practice what I and so many celebrities know and practice. My goal is to democratize health: to make health accessible to everyone, no matter who. Whether you live in New York, Nebraska, or Nevada; no matter how much money you make; no matter what your natural build is or your genetic predispositions are; no matter what your social status, job, race, nationality, or sexual preference may be; no matter what foods you love or hate; no matter how much you like or don't like to exercise; no matter whether your appearance is important for your career or not; no matter how you feel today when you look in the mirror—if you are sick of obsessing and beating yourself up about food and weight, this book is for you.

I am a "health foodie" because I love good, high-quality, natural foods that makes me feel better, stronger, and more energized. However, when I cook, taste is just as important to me as nutritional content. Regardless of how healthful a food is, nobody will want to eat it if it doesn't taste good, and I believe food is meant to be enjoyed, not just tolerated. For me, "good enough" is never good enough when it comes to food (or anything, for that matter!). If you don't enjoy food, why bother? I don't believe in eating mediocre food just because it will supposedly make you thinner. *It won't*. We should all know that by now.

To me, food that doesn't taste delicious is worthless. On the other hand, I'm not interested in eating high-fat, high-sugar foods with no fiber, vitamins, or minerals. Sometimes I do eat processed food, but this is more the exception than the rule. I'm not interested in highly processed food or food that might taste good for a minute but doesn't do anything for my health. It's a balance. I consider my daily diet my bank account, with calories I have to manage—and I'll tell you more about that in Chapter 1.

Before we get to the ten rules I've created for becoming naturally thin, you might want to know something about me. A lot of what I know about food comes from a natural passion for both food and health. I grew up eating every meal in a restaurant, and my proclivity toward healthy living has grown out of an unstable upbringing that inspired me to take control of my own life and make something good out of it. This has been a long progression for me: to rise up out of a difficult childhood that set me up for a lot of unhealthy attitudes about food; to embrace a more real, natural, balanced way of cooking, eating, and looking at the world. Today, I eat and live as a naturally thin person, but it has been a journey.

That journey, fueled by my passion for food and health, led me to the National Gourmet Institute for Health and Culinary Arts in 2000. I spent a year at this school, and although I originally went there for fun, I was soon hooked on the chef's life and on new ideas for making the most out of good food. But what I did with my education is a little different from what most of my classmates did. I didn't go on to work in a restaurant. I wanted to do something bigger, something that would reach more people.

One thing I did was to start my own line of low-fat, low-calorie, dairy-free, wheat-free, egg-free baked goods, called BethennyBakes™, in 2001. I was a contestant on *Martha Stewart: Apprentice* and people referred to me as the breakout star on that show. (I'll tell you more about that experience later.) I have cooked for celebrities such as Alicia Silverstone, Denis Leary, and Mariska Hargitay. I've been featured on morning shows, including the *Today* show, CBS's *The Early Show*, and *Good Day New York*, talking about healthy cooking and eating; and I've appeared on other shows, too, such as *Access Hollywood*, *Entertainment Tonight*, and *Extra*. I write a regular column for *Health* magazine, and I've written for or been written about in the *New York Times*, *People*, *InStyle*, *Family Circle*, *Hamptons*, *OK!* magazine, *Ladies Home Journal*, *USA Today*, *US Weekly*, *TV Guide*, and the *Wall Street Journal*, among many others. My cooking videos get thousands of hits on YouTube.com, and I have been a spokesperson for brands including Pepperidge Farms Baked Naturals Snacks, Cascade, and Tupperware. I recently finished filming the second season of *The Real Housewives of New York City*. And now, I've written this book.

What I know, and what I've learned over the course of my life, about getting and staying thin isn't just a matter of healthful, delicious food (although that is a big part of the picture). I've also learned a lot about how to *think* about food, how to *balance* diet with the rest of life, and how to stop torturing myself about every mouthful. When you live in New York City, it's difficult not to be obsessed with appearance, food, and dieting. But I realize it's difficult not to be obsessed with appearances, food, and dieting no matter where you live. If you share this struggle, then we have something very important in common, and I want to help you win.

I'm naturally thin, but I didn't come preprogrammed that way. I arrived there by changing my habits and learning how to think like a naturally thin person. The result: I became a naturally thin person, one of those people you looked at in high school and wondered how they did it. Amazingly enough, it was easy—a lot easier than my diet-obsessed self would have ever dreamed. Back when I was burdened, overwhelmed, and ingrained with the diet mentality, I never really thought I could escape. But I did.

I can't believe how much of my life I've wasted feeling anxious, depressed, antisocial, and—after binging on something—full of self-loathing because my jeans were too tight. I can't believe how much of my life I wasted *feeling fat,* obsessing about what to order on a date or how to get out of an invitation to a restaurant I perceived as serving fattening food. Does that sound familiar? Do you feel full of regret every time you eat something that doesn't fit your perception of diet food? Have food, fat, carbs, and dieting created such a level of anxiety and preoccupation in your life that you think about them all day long? Been there, done that—but I'm not there and I don't ever do that anymore. Why not join me in this new state of mind?

Guess what happened when I escaped from this kind of thinking. I got thin, for life. I can't even imagine going back to my old ways of thinking, eating, and behaving—my *heavy habits,* those habits that perpetuated my self-destructive thinking and eating. (I'll talk more about heavy habits later in this book.) I broke free, and now I have *thin thoughts*. And you can, too, no matter who you are.

The greatest gift I can give you, and the greatest gift you can give yourself, is *Naturally Thin*. I've condensed everything I've learned about eating and cooking into ten simple rules you can use to change your own *heavy habits,* your own thinking, your body, your energy level, your health, your whole life. Think you've heard these tips before? Think again—this book doesn't tell you what to eat. Instead, I show you how to change your life without changing who you are, what you like, or how you live. I show you how to change your habits and the way you think about food, no matter what you like to eat or how you like to live, because that's where your body starts—in your head.

Diets Don't Work

You might have heard this before, and dismissed it as a line. But it's not a line. It's true. Some people define insanity as repeating the same behavior and expecting different results every time. Are we all crazy? How many diets have you started? How much money have you spent feeding the diet industry? Have you lost weight, strayed from the diet, and gained back all the weight (and more)? Of course you have. We all have. And yet, we keep going on to the next "new" diet, the one that promises to finally fix our weight problems. It never does. What's *wrong* with us?

Life is too short to waste obsessing over fat grams or carb grams or never, ever exceeding 1,200 calories a day. How many ounces of that cereal should you eat? Is your steak bigger than a deck of cards? Is your serving of rice larger than your fist? Is that two ounces of pasta on your plate, or are you "binging" on three ounces? Come on. It's ridiculous and obsessive.

It's amazing how many highly intelligent people can be so uninformed when dealing with food, and so stuck in harmful ruts they don't even realize they are in. How many times have your conversations at a dinner or a cocktail party revolved around somebody's saying, "Oh, you should only eat steak; it's a miracle diet" or "You have to try the cabbage soup diet; it's amazing"? Diet talk is common at social events, and people talk as if they were authorities on whatever their latest plan is—but at the next party, you find out that they are off the wagon or are pushing something else. How many times have people told you they are "starting a new diet tomorrow"? Or maybe you are the one who has been saying this to other people.

How many of those people have lost a lot of weight and kept it off for good?

The simple fact is that you don't function normally if you constantly have to measure, count, restrict, and obsess over food. You feel punished, deprived, even angry. I know I did. Eventually, life intervenes, and you no longer have time or patience for all that nonsense. Then you give up and tell yourself, "Well, I might as well just eat the whole double cheese pizza because dieting is just too hard."

Of course it's hard. It's not natural to eat like that, and it's not healthy, either—not physically, not mentally. If you have to rely on a regimen, a menu, strict rules, or even a book to tell you what to do and what to eat, you aren't going to stick with it. You don't need something to control your life. You just need some tools that will help *you* regain control. After all, it's your body. You can change it if you want to change it.

Notice that I *don't* say you are going to need willpower. I say *control* because that's exactly what I mean. You are your own person. You are in control of what you do. You have the power. It's your body, your life, your mind, *your food*. You have control over what you choose to do and how you choose to act. The problem with diets is that they give you the idea that someone else is controlling you: a famous guy tells a famous girl what to eat; or a diet plan somebody wrote for you tells you how many cups of this and how many tablespoons of that you can eat.

Frankly, this lets you off the hook. If you are on a diet, the diet controls you, so when things go wrong, you can blame the diet. If you are on a diet, you don't have to take responsibility for your own life. The diet tells you what to do, and if it doesn't work, you hate the diet; the diet failed; you are the victim. Even as you feel guilty and blame yourself for your inner weakness, deep down, you don't feel that you've ever been the one at the steering wheel. The diet has been driving. You're just along for the ride. And that's no way to live your life.

Take back the wheel and start driving yourself through life again. Sure, taking back your life can be a challenge, but getting *naturally thin* is easier than you think. This book is about *you* and the ways *you* can learn to deal, face-to-face, with food again, rather than letting food deal with *you*.

More about Me

I wouldn't describe my childhood as typical, but I would describe it as challenging. I grew up moving from place to place. I was a bicoastal child, going back and forth from New York to Los Angeles until the age of six, then living all over the place. In New York, we lived in Manhattan, Forest Hills, Rockville Centre, Old Westbury, and Locust Valley. We also lived in Boston, Florida, and Los Angeles. I went to thirteen different schools. I had no stability whatsoever, no structure, no regular meals, and nothing to instill a healthy attitude about food. I ate almost all my meals in restaurants.

My mother loved and hated food at the same time. At least, that's how it seemed to me, and I think her bad habits inspired me to develop a healthier lifestyle, so I could be different than she was. But her food obsessions also stuck to me. I admit I am a type A person who tends to get a bit obsessive about things, and I've spent plenty of years of my life obsessing about food and working hard to be thin. In fact, I've been watching my weight since grade school. My mother's father instilled in her that fat wasn't an option, so my mother was just passing along a family tradition when she instilled these food attitudes in me.

As for my father, he was never really around. He was a horse trainer, as was my stepfather, so I spent a lot of time at the track as a kid. That wasn't such a great example. I started visiting the betting window at age six. In many ways, I had to raise myself. That made developing a healthy ego pretty tough.

Like a lot of kids, I had a chubby adolescent phase, but unlike a lot of mothers, my mother took me to an obesity clinic when I was nine. It was immediately clear to me that gaining weight was *not* acceptable. For years afterward, my weight fluctuated, but *dieting* was always in the forefront of my mind, from an early age. I remember my mother seeing an overweight girl and commenting that if this were her child, she would lock the girl in a closet and send in water on a tray. That made an impression on me, even though I knew she was joking (sort of). Being fat wasn't an option.

At the same time, we were always eating in restaurants or getting takeout Chinese food or pizza. In other words, my mother rarely cooked. The only meals I remember that seemed home-prepared were the bagels we ate every Sunday morning. I was eating escargots by the age of four. Kids' menu? I never knew such a thing existed.

I loved food. And yet, I also feared it. By the age of ten, I already knew all about the Beverly Hills Diet. I obsessed about food, and pushed it away, too. I remember ripping out the diet pages in magazines from a very young age; and over the years, I've tried all the diets. The Beverly Hills Diet, the Eat Your Weight in Fruit Diet, the Cabbage Soup Diet, the Atkins Diet, the South Beach Diet, Weight-Watchers, Jenny Craig, NutriSystem, the Flight Attendant's Diet (at the time, it was called the Stewardess Diet), the Grapefruit Diet, Slim-Fast, the Zone, Diet Center, Diet Designs, the Raw Food Diet, and every other diet I happened to run across in a magazine.

I like to think of myself as an intelligent person, and yet I kept on dieting. It was a way of life, one that I inherited from my mother, and one that she inherited from her father, who also made sure she understood that being fat was not an option.

I don't blame my mother, my grandfather, or even my father, for my attitudes toward and my struggles with dieting, body image, and food. I don't even blame the magazines, books, and movies that conveyed impossible images of beauty and the supposed necessity of constant dieting. We are all smart enough to know it's not necessarily realistic to weigh 105 pounds. Yes, we are all, to some extent, products of our parents' unresolved issues, but I truly believe most people do the best they can. We are all fighting against our own issues, and food and diet were my issues. I'm guessing that if you are reading this book, they are your issues, too.

When I became an adult, my love of fine food led me to cooking school, but my attitudes toward food really started to change on one of my trips to Italy. As a chef, I vowed not to miss any food experiences in the country with the most amazing food in the world.

I vowed not to obsess about every calorie and not to miss out on cappuccino, pasta, great wine, and wonderful desserts. But in Italy, I discovered something much more important than good food. I discovered a new attitude.

In general, Europeans view food and eating differently than Americans. They value food more than Americans do, but obsess about it less. That was a revelation to me, especially when I saw beautiful, naturally thin Italians eating anything they wanted. I began to shift my perspective. I began to understand how to enjoy food—any food—and still be *naturally thin*.

When I came back from Italy, changed but without having gained an ounce, I began to refine and crystallize the lessons I had absorbed. The result is this book. The lessons I've learned over the years have served me well because my life is extremely fast-paced and stressful. It would be easy for me to continue my unhealthy habits, from starving myself to binge eating. But I don't.

When I filmed *Martha Stewart: Apprentice*, I had just gotten over pneumonia. Being on a competition reality show is brutal, unbelievably stressful, and exhausting, and what was everybody else living on? Energy drinks and meal replacement bars. But not me. During the entire filming of that show, I took the time to make myself three meals a day, no matter what else was going on. I ate healthful food nobody else was eating—because I know that it takes only five minutes to make, for example, a veggie sandwich or turkey on wholegrain bread.

Everybody has five minutes. That's the only reason I got through the experience with my health and sanity intact—and I'm not kidding. I was healthy going into the experience because of my new way of life, and that by itself was significant in getting me through. I knew if I was eating processed food—or, worse, eating food from the street vendors—I wouldn't make it. When you are on a reality show, you want comfort food, but energy drinks and hot dogs aren't going to provide real comfort. You get very little sleep, or you don't sleep at all. You have cravings because you are under stress, and when you aren't sleeping, you are running around like a maniac. Eating well was an important investment for me during that time—and is still important, every day of my life.

Filming *The Real Housewives of New York City* has been incredibly grueling, too. My entire life is right there, on camera, for everyone to see. As we filmed our second season, I found myself with very little time to spare, let alone time to eat well. But this is my life and I accept and welcome all my challenges. My positive mentality has affected everyone around me. The other housewives are losing weight, and all my friends have lost weight. Being *naturally thin* has radiated out to everyone I know. It's amazing.

Your life is probably a little or a lot different from mine, but you probably also have stress, a grueling schedule, and very little time to eat well. I understand. But know that you can still be *naturally thin, without dieting,* no matter what your life is like. Today, I'm a thirty-something woman living in New York City, and I no longer diet. I eat pretty much whatever I want to eat. And for the first time in my life, my weight is completely and surprisingly consistent. I look and feel better than I ever did before. I'm in charge. I'm not a doctor, I'm not a nutritionist, and I'm not a fitness expert. And, most important, I am *not* in charge of *you.* But I am a natural foods chef, a dedicated lover of delicious food, and a healthy, thin person. I'm also a person who wants to tell you how I broke the code, broke through the chains of dieting, and learned how to incorporate the ten simple rules into my own life.

I admit that I have an advantage, living in New York, where I can experience an impressive culinary variety. But this can also be a disadvantage. I could easily spend my days eating honey-roasted nuts, hot pretzels, and hot dogs. Every deli on the street has ice cream, pizza, burgers, and salad bars. In the City that Never Sleeps, it's easy to eat too much at any hour of the day or night. It's a world of variety, and also a world of temptation.

Even if you don't live in a big city, you have similar challenges. In New York, we have to go to six different markets to get the things we need to cook a meal. You might have access to a mega-mart with everything you need—and plenty of tempting things you don't need.

The New York Greenmarkets are fantastic, but you probably have farmers' markets and produce stands near you. Maybe you think you can't afford to eat well and fast food is your only option, but that's not true, either. This book will show you lots of great ways to eat well economically. Maybe you are a soccer mom continually tempted by the ice cream truck, your kids' leftovers, and pizza deliveries, but what about the girl in the city who lives right above the all-night pizza place? You have challenges. We all do. We are all different. But we can all be *naturally thin*.

No matter where you live, you can find and prepare good food. You don't have to settle for processed, packaged food that doesn't thrill or even satisfy you. You don't have to live on drive-through food or convenience food. You can eat just as well as I eat, and just as well as celebrities eat.

This is exactly what I want to do for you. I want to counsel and guide you, the same way I guide my friends and the celebrities who ask me for advice. Why should celebrities be the only ones to benefit from the secrets I've learned? You're busy, just as they are. You want to look fantastic, just as they do. You might not be on a set, filming a new blockbuster movie, but that doesn't mean you don't need energy and healthful meals that fit into your packed schedule. You might not be wearing vintage Chanel to the Academy Awards ceremony, but that doesn't mean you don't want to look drop-dead gorgeous in your new dress. The paparazzi may not be stalking you to see what you eat, but your friends notice. Your kids notice, too. What kind of example are you setting?

As you can probably tell, I've replaced my dieting obsession with an obsession for cooking and eating the very best food, and sharing it with everyone. I've already shared these secrets with my friends, and they have all benefited. Now it's your turn. It's my obsession to help everyone who wants to be *naturally thin* achieve what I have achieved. That's just the way I am. I have to obsess about something. The point is that this obsession is all about feeling and looking great—for me, for the rich and famous, and for *you*.

It's also about finally getting rid of all the extra weight you've been carrying around—the weight you don't need. That weight is holding you back from being your true self, and the only way to find your true self is to embrace healthful eating as a way of life. You can't do it by suffering, deprivation, or pain. You can't do it by starving or binging and purging. And you don't have to do any of that anymore.

Healthful eating is something worth getting excited about. All you have to do is work through the ten rules. Read them; practice the tips for incorporating them into your life; and slowly but surely, you'll see your life, your attitude, and your body changing, right before your eyes. Start practicing now, and in just days you'll feel more like yourself again. I'm ready to help you transform your entire relationship to food, exactly the way I help my clients change theirs. Are you ready?

What to Expect inside This Book

This book will teach you a new language and a new mind set. I've divided this book into two parts. In Part One, I talk about the ten rules I've learned for getting and staying *naturally thin*. I devote one chapter to each rule, explaining it in depth so that you will understand what I mean and how to incorporate the rule into your life. I'll talk about how each rule works for me, and how it can work for you. Memorize these rules and live them, and you'll start to see exactly how easy it is to be naturally thin.

I suggest you take your time with Part One. Let it sink in. Think about it, read it, and read it again. Go back over the sections that speak to you, and I'll be with you the whole way, sharing my own struggles and helping you manage yours. The more you think about and practice the ten rules, the more they will become integrated into your consciousness. Before you know it, you'll be practicing them without even thinking. They will become part of who you are and how you think about food. And starting with the very first chapter, you'll be able to stop dieting, stop obsessing about food, and stop wrecking your own happiness and health. You'll be free—and you'll start getting thinner.

Part Two of this book is for people who want more structure. Make no mistake: this is not a diet. But it does offer some solid guidelines for how to implement the rules in your life. In Chapter 11, I set up some principles for you to practice and I also review the ten rules. I talk about some important concepts and remind you of others from Part One. Then I take your hand and lead you through a week of eating.

During the chapters on the week of eating, I talk about a lot of things, from what to eat for breakfast, lunch, and dinner to handling special occasions, travel, and cooking at home. What do you do when faced with a gigantic muffin at Starbucks? What do you do when you have to find a meal at a convenience store? How do you handle a breakfast buffet without panicking or gaining ten pounds in one sitting? What do you do about happy hour? It's all covered here.

I also tell you, throughout Part Two, exactly what I am eating for each meal on each day of the week. This information will be in boxes called "Bethenny Bytes," because they are bytes of information about my personal food choices. But these boxes are not meant to tell *you* what to eat. In fact, sometimes I set a really bad example! The point is to show you that *naturally thin* people live normal lives and face normal challenges, and knowing how to face them—including how to feel when you make bad choices or eat too much—is the heart of the matter.

Throughout the entire book, you'll notice a couple of features. Some boxes highlight "Naturally Thin Thoughts," which are tips to help you correct your thinking. Other boxes highlight "Heavy Habits," the bad habits you have and the destructive things you might be thinking, and what you can do about them. Finally, I'll occasionally include "Celebrity Secrets" boxes, with stories about celebrities. Some of these celebrities have been my clients; others I've just met. How they eat can be helpful to you, both as good examples and as not-so-great examples. Some celebrities have great habits. Others are still saddled with dieting. Many of them are a lot like you.

Most of the chapters in this book also include recipes at the end. I need to make a point here about the recipes. I'm not a measurer. This drove my teachers in cooking school crazy because they wanted to know exactly how much of this or that I put into something I made. But even if I could not tell them this, I could always make the recipe again. Although I have some measurements in my recipes, they are really not very precise. My style of writing recipes is fairly casual, too. So I'd like you to view the recipes in this book as guidelines. Feel free to be creative and stray from them, or replace some ingredients with others that you like better. I'm all about experimenting and exploring the world of taste and flavor, so I encourage you to enter your own kitchen with that same adventurous spirit. For more recipes, be sure to look for my *Naturally Thin* cookbook, due out next year.

Come with me through this book. I've got so much to tell you, and I'm so excited to help you find the peace, the truth, and the freedom I've found. I promise you, it's not going to be unpleasant. It's going to be fun, enlightening, even delicious. You're going to learn how to enjoy your food again, guilt-free. You're going to drop the extra weight you've been carrying around. Best of all, you're going to feel better than you've ever felt in your life. You're going to be *naturally thin*.

Part One

THE RULES

Chapter 1

YOUR DIET
IS A BANK ACCOUNT

It's Your Right to Be Thin

If you've read the introduction to this book, or if you've seen me on television or watched any of my videos about healthful cooking, you probably already know that, having become a naturally thin person I have a mission: to *democratize health*. I cook for celebrities and advise my friends about healthy eating, but why should celebrities and my friends get all the benefits? Celebrities often have jobs that require them to look great, but this doesn't mean you can't be privy to their secrets. They don't all belong to some secret "thin club" that you don't belong to. You belong to this club, too. You just haven't filled out your membership card yet.

I think everybody deserves to be healthy and get into the best shape of her life. That's why I've collected all the simple facts that have taken me twenty years to learn, and crystallized them into ten simple rules. Now I'm going to hand them to you.

You can be naturally thin. I don't care what your body type, blood type, or personality type is. I don't care how much your mom weighs, or what food you just can't live without. Look, even celebrities like Oprah Winfrey and Britney Spears have a hard time keeping weight off, despite all their diet coaches and personal trainers, but they haven't yet figured out what it means to be naturally thin.

I spent twenty years suffering through diet hell before I finally figured out that being naturally thin has nothing to do with having a fast metabolism or certain genetics or anything else you can't control. I'm in my mid-thirties now, and I'm thinner than I was in my twenties. People ask me if I crash-diet, or they say, "Oh, you're just naturally thin." It's true, I am naturally thin—now. But it wasn't always that way.

Millions of women get caught up in the insane cycle of dieting, failing, and dieting again. Well, it's time to cut it out. No more diets. Do you understand me? *Stop dieting now.*

That probably sounds like an impossibly wonderful idea to some of you. A few months ago, one of my girlfriends said to me, "You know what? I'm done. I am so sick of dieting and exercising. I can't do it anymore." I remember being in that same place, and if you picked up this book, you probably know that same feeling.

So do it. Step up right now and take possession of your right to be thin. You are an adult. It's time to stop letting somebody else tell you what to eat, how to eat, or why to eat. Forget it. Kick out the tyrannical chauffeur in your life, whose name is "diet," and slide into that driver's seat. You're in charge. The suffering stops now.

Rule 1: Your Diet Is a Bank Account

Let's get right to the first rule. I consider this a sort of master rule, the mother of all the other rules. It's the first thing I tell people when they ask me how I stay naturally thin. Every rule is important—even crucial—but this rule encompasses all the others. It's something I keep in mind every day, every time I eat anything. It has become a part of my life to think about and implement this rule, and it makes the whole thing so simple and sensible, you won't believe that you've never practiced it. Here it is:

NATURALLY THIN THOUGHT

So you love chocolate or cheese? Or you hate to exercise? No problem. Lots of naturally thin people share those same preferences. You can still be *you*, no matter who you are, *and* be naturally thin. If you don't eat what you want to eat, if you restrict yourself, you will feel deprived, and it will all fall apart eventually. You won't keep it up. Eat what you want to eat. Just recognize what you are eating, and if you know it's an "expensive" investment, enjoy every bite—but have only a couple of bites. Or just recognize and balance it later. Then you won't blow your budget and you can stay balanced. If you hate to exercise, you eat a little less. If you love to exercise, you can eat a little more. Balance.

Your diet is a bank account.

This is the first thing I want you to think about every day, and start to integrate into your life. Until it becomes second nature, you need to keep reminding yourself: *Your diet is a bank account.*

Just as you balance your spending and savings, you must balance your food choices. Don't eat too much of any one thing, don't eat the same thing twice, balance starches with proteins, vegetables and fruits with sweets, and always balance a splurge with a save. This balancing is approximate—but it works, and it works without counting, measuring, or obsessing.

Most of the time—on most days and for most meals and snacks—make *smart investments* in healthful foods that fill you up. Then, when you really want to splurge, go ahead. You aren't dieting, remember. You are living. *However,* a splurge comes with a price. You have to balance that splurge by cutting back a little afterward, until your accounts are in order again. It's that simple.

Do you really want to throw away your calories on something you don't like? That's like spending money on something you'll never use or something that doesn't fit. It's a waste. Make smart investments that will be good for your body and will make you feel better. That makes a worthwhile splurge perfectly reasonable. When it's not so worthwhile, save up those calories for later. That's sound bank-account management.

Sure, just like financial independence, dietary balance can sometimes be challenging. If you've been overeating and not balancing your food choices for a few years now, you probably have some excess weight. This weight is like debt. But you can pay off debt and get rid of extra weight in just the same way—a little at a time. Chip away at that weight by daily balancing, but don't obsess by budgeting every penny and counting every calorie. You can achieve your ideal body weight—financial independence. Eat a lot here; eat less there. Eat less here; eat more later.

HEAVY HABIT

Have you ever thought to yourself, *I ate too much, I ruined it, so I might as well just keep eating*? Then you go on a tear because you've given up hope. Do you know that feeling? I compare this to buyer's remorse. If you indulge in something, then sit up all night feeling guilty about it, you won't be in any position to make balanced choices. You'll just make it worse for yourself. The other day, one of my friends called me and said, "I ruined myself, I'm ruined. I ate five cookies." I remember that feeling—but I don't have it anymore. I eat, but I don't let guilt and remorse spur me on to a binge. Sometimes, I eat too much. But then I pick myself up and brush myself off. Instead of making this a reason to eat even more (where is the logic in that?), I remember: *Your diet is a bank account.*

Bank Account Balancing How-Tos

This all sounds great in theory, I know. But how do you actually do it? Stay conscious of what you eat, and make conscious decisions about it. Food is not in charge. You are, so take charge and decide in a rational and conscious way what to eat.

Let's say you had pancakes for breakfast. They're fine—and starchy and sweet. So what do you have for lunch? Pasta? Of course not. That's more starch. You are balancing your diet like a bank account now, so you know that because you had starch and sugar earlier in the day, now, you need protein and vegetables. So have a salad with grilled chicken or some vegetable soup. Or maybe you had eggs for breakfast. No problem. Pasta or a sandwich might be just the thing for lunch, or dinner. Balance your proteins with your starches; balance your fruits and vegetables with your sweets and fats.

Never have the same kind of food for two meals in a row. Get a little of everything, but not too much of anything.

Balancing also applies to amounts. If you have a really light breakfast, you can have a little more for lunch. If you had a really big lunch, go light on dinner. If you ate a lot all day one day, go easy the next day. Just stay tuned in to what you are doing, and you'll be able to have the foods you really love—in a balanced way. This is how naturally thin people eat—without deprivation, without dieting, but in balance. Once you get into the habit, it's easier than you think. Practice this for a few days and you will start to become naturally aware, honing your instincts about what your body needs and wants. When you become the fine-tuned machine that you are going to become, you will instinctively know what the next meal should be. You'll know how to handle any food situation.

In Part Two of this book, I'll go more into incorporating this rule into your daily life. But first, let's consider some of the surprising obstacles you may find in your path, as well as some tools to help you.

NATURALLY THIN THOUGHT

Balancing is not about counting calories, fat grams, carbs, or anything else. Don't bother with this, because you won't keep up with it. It takes too much time, and you are too busy. Besides, it is obsessive, and you don't want to go there. Instead, you just need to *pay attention*, and tap into your common sense. This balancing is approximate, but it works. Just keep it in your head. The calories will work themselves out. Now it's not obsessive; it's not food noise. You know what to eat. Just listen to your food voice.

Your Food Noise, Your Food Voice

Balancing your account is crucial to becoming naturally thin, but it isn't the only factor. You've got other things going on inside your head, I know. So let's talk about those things because they can become hurdles or tools, getting in your way or helping you succeed. Let's talk about your *food noise*, and your *food voice*.

Food noise is your negative inner food dialogue, commenting on and criticizing everything you eat, or think about eating, or don't eat. Food noise yammers at you about how you screwed up when you ate that pasta. Food noise berates you for eyeing that cheesecake or for not going to the gym today. Food noise reminds you what that number on the scale said this morning, and yells it in your ear all day long, making you feel bad—or good, if you lost a few pounds, as if a two-pound water-weight loss makes you a better person. Food noise makes you focus on the body parts you hate, and makes you feel powerless to change anything. Food noise is mean. Food noise makes you feel bad.

Food noise is a product of the past, as well as of current stress and anxiety. Did you grow up learning that food equals love? Do you use food to comfort yourself or calm yourself down when you are stressed? Does a bad day mean you *deserve* to eat the whole pizza?

Do you think you won't ever be thin, so why even try? Food noise tells each person something different, but you need to recognize *your* food noise for what it is, so that you can stop dignifying it with a response.

There is an antidote for food noise. If your food noise is the little devil on your left shoulder that tells you to eat a cheeseburger just because you saw one on a television commercial, your *food voice* is the little angel on your right shoulder that has the real information about whether you actually *want* a cheeseburger or not. Your food noise is based on the past, but your food voice always looks to the future. Your food voice tells you what you really, truly want and need. It isn't just the voice that reminds you that you haven't had any protein yet today and you really need some (although your food voice will do this for you). It's also the voice that says: *Wait a minute. I don't really like these fat-free cookies. I want a real cookie. Is that so wrong?* (Of course it isn't.) That is your food voice.

Your food voice is your body's organic sense of itself. *Right inside you*, you have all the information you need to be naturally thin. Your food voice might be hoarse by now, yelling at you because you aren't listening, giving you all kinds of signals, showing you that you are making choices that aren't right for you; but if your food voice is getting drowned out by your food noise, you may suffer from indigestion, hunger pains, sore joints, headache, feeling tired, or feeling low on energy. Hello! This is your food voice talking! It's trying to get your attention.

If you can just start to listen, you will quickly learn that your food voice has wonderful things to tell you. It makes you feel great when you make smart food investments. It tells you what to eat based on what your body really wants, and it tells you when you've had enough, too. Your food voice is nice to you. It makes you feel good.

Especially for those of us who have trouble distinguishing between our food noise and our food voice—and for those whose food noise drowns out the food voice completely—treating your diet like a bank account is an absolutely essential step to helping sort out the confusion.

> **NATURALLY THIN THOUGHT**
>
> Have you ever noticed that sometimes you'll eat something decadent and in-dulgent and feel really awful, bloated, and guilty; but at other times you'll eat something decadent and indulgent and you'll feel great, practically buzzing with happiness? That's your food voice. It tells you when you are eating because you really need *or want* something, rather than just eating for the sake of eating. And (this is important), it also tells you when to *stop eating*.

All bodies seek balance, so when you purposefully and system-atically integrate a balancing mechanism into your life—balancing your diet like a bank account and following the other rules in this book—your food voice will automatically get stronger and more confident. Your food noise, taken aback, might just learn to shut up a little. Balancing your diet like a bank account is a training exer-cise, and although it might sound a bit difficult at first, it quickly be-comes second nature. Your body wants you to do this, so everything will start to fall in place when you do.

The Differential

I have a few more tools for you. Another very important con-cept to understand as you balance your splurges and your savings is something I call the *differential*. I'll be using this term frequently throughout the book, so let's talk about it right now, and about what it means.

The *differential* is the difference between two choices, and whether or not that difference is worthwhile. Here's an example. I love chili because of the flavors and textures: the chili powder, cumin, toma-toes, peppers, and beans. But there are a lot of kinds of chili out there—beef chili, turkey chili, veggie chili. To me, the *differential* between a fatty, beef-filled chili and turkey or veggie chili is nothing. I often can't even tell the difference. So in the case of chili, it's definitely worth it for me to make the lighter, healthier choice.

But here's where the *differential* is big for me: give me a choice between a fatty New York strip steak topped with butter and a bland poached chicken breast. To me, that's a huge *differential*. I love the fatty steak; I admit it. I get so much pleasure out of this food that it's not worth it to me to choose the chicken breast. I saved elsewhere, when it didn't matter so much, in order to get the full pleasure of the New York strip steak experience. That being said, I usually eat only a few bites. If I eat the skinless chicken breast, I'll eat the whole thing and still be bored and longing for something more; by contrast, I can have a few amazing bites of the steak and be completely satisfied. I would rather have three delicious bites of fatty steak than four times as much boring chicken. This is a quality vs. quantity concept.

Of course, choosing the more decadent option comes with a price. We aren't living in an alternative reality where unlimited amounts of white sugar or beef fat have no impact on your waistline or health. As a natural foods chef, I know perfectly well that I should not be eating fatty steak every day, and when I do eat it, I shouldn't eat very much of it. I know I should really limit how much I eat. So I have a few delicious bites. Then, I stop. Most of my meal will consist of other healthy foods I love, like salad and sautéed vegetables. I fill up on these first, but I also refuse to deny myself the pleasure of those bites of steak.

Your *differential* will probably be different from mine when you apply it to any given food. Maybe you hate the fatty steak and a nicely seasoned grilled piece of light fish or tofu is just as satisfying as, if not more satisfying than, fatty steak. That's great. Make the healthier choice, and save your fat and calorie allowance for something that matters more to you, like crème brûlée or french fries. In this book I am not going to tell you to eat whatever I eat, because I want you to understand, appreciate, and really get to know *your own true preferences*. This is balancing your account.

The Point of Diminishing Returns

Another concept I'll talk about throughout this book is the *point of diminishing returns*. This concept is also closely related to balancing your diet like a bank account, because this is the concept that allows you to monitor your food "spending" and know when to stop.

The *point of diminishing returns* is what I call that point when a bite you take isn't quite as good as the bite before it. For example, let's say you really love fried calamari. You have a bite, and it is out of this world. You are tasting and enjoying your splurge. The next bite might be just as good. The third bite, though? Maybe the enjoyment level has peaked, and while the calamari still tastes good, that third bite isn't quite as amazing as the first two. Instead of just plowing through the rest of the plate, stop at the *point of diminishing returns*.

Why keep eating it and adding more calories to your bank account? It's never going to get any better. Anything after that is just a waste of calories. You laughed; you cried; it was better than *Cats*. Now it's over, so stop eating and move on with your life.

This balancing act, this idea of a bank account, is not a miracle cure that will banish twenty pounds in two days. *This is not a diet.*

NATURALLY THIN THOUGHT

I've cooked for a lot of people with a lot of different diets they want to or have to follow—vegan, low-carb, gluten-free, kosher, all-natural, organic, or whatever it might be. Because this book isn't about a diet, it works with any special dietary restrictions you might have. You can follow the ten rules in this book no matter what you eat. You can always balance your diet like a bank account. Whether you can't eat wheat or choose not to eat meat, balance your choices and you'll feel better.

This is a gentle, long-term recalibration of your thoughts and a new vernacular, a new attitude about food that will free you from dieting. Being naturally thin is a journey and a process that start now. You won't be deprived and you won't be giving up anything except some extra weight. So why waste another minute?

Rule 1 Recipes

To get yourself on track and in balancing mode, try these recipes. Denis Leary loves this stuffed mushroom recipe; it's one of the ways I got him to eat more vegetables. If you have a sweet tooth, whip up these Banana Oatmeal Chocolate Chip Cookies, for a light and satisfying sweet snack.

Stuffed Portobello Mushrooms

Denis loves these stuffed mushrooms. They helped convince him that vegetables really can be delicious.

Serves 4

4 large portobello mushrooms

1 clove garlic, minced

Store-bought balsamic vinaigrette dressing

1 teaspoon Dijon mustard

Salt and pepper, to taste

1 tablespoon chopped parsley

4–5 button mushrooms, chopped

¼ cup Parmesan cheese

2 tablespoons toasted pine nuts (lightly toast in a small nonstick pan on medium heat, watch carefully, as they burn quickly)

Additional 1 tablespoon Parmesan and 1 teaspoon chopped parsley

1. Wipe portobellos clean with a damp paper towel. Do not rinse! Remove large stems. Cut off hard base and finely chop the remaining

stem, then set aside. Mix garlic, balsamic dressing, Dijon mustard, and salt and pepper in a bowl. Using a brush, generously brush the entire mushroom cap with the marinade. Place mushrooms in a ziplock bag and refrigerate for no less than 1 hour.

2. Preheat oven to 400°F. Combine parsley, button mushrooms, and Parmesan. Taste mixture and season with salt and pepper.

3. Grill mushroom caps on an outdoor grill or in a grill pan or non-stick skillet. During the grilling, place a pan or some sort of weight on top of the mushrooms. This will make them crispier and remove some of the water. Grill until lightly charred, then flip and repeat. Place mushrooms on tinfoil or a sheet pan, spread the mushroom stem mixture on top of each portobello, sprinkle with pine nuts and additional Parmesan, and bake for 10 minutes. For the last 5 minutes, place under the broiler. Sprinkle with additional parsley and serve.

Banana Oatmeal Chocolate Chip Cookies

These are one of my faves, and one of Susan Sarandon's, too. It's a cute story, how we met. I met Susan Sarandon at a red-carpet event. She complimented me on my necklace, which Sheryl Crow had admired at a Rolling Stones concert a few weeks earlier. I had another necklace like it in my purse to give to Sheryl, so I laughed and said, "I have one in my purse for Sheryl Crow. Do you want one, too?" I felt like one of those guys on the street saying, "Hey, want to buy a watch?" I told her I would send her one, and she just smiled and said, "No, you won't." But I got the contact info for her agent and I did send her one, along with some of my BethennyBakes Banana Oatmeal Cookies. Now I send her cookies on a regular basis.

Serves 10 cookies

1½ cups oat flour
¾ cup rolled oats
½ teaspoon baking powder
½ teaspoon baking soda
½ teaspoon salt
½ cup raw sugar

⅓ cup chocolate chips

1 teaspoon canola oil

⅓ cup soymilk

½ cup banana puree (1 medium-size banana)

1 teaspoon vanilla extract

1. Preheat oven to 375°F. Combine all the dry ingredients in a bowl. Combine all the wet ingredients in a separate bowl. Mix the dry and wet ingredients together, until well combined.

2. Use a medium-size ice cream scoop or a large spoon to scoop batter onto a cookie sheet covered with wax paper. Bake for 12 minutes, rotating the pan halfway through cooking, or bake until the edges of the cookies are light brown.

Chapter 2

YOU CAN HAVE IT ALL, JUST NOT ALL AT ONCE

Now that you are thinking in terms of balancing your diet like a bank account, you are ready for the second rule. This rule sounds a little like something you would say to a two-year-old, but for some of us, that's as far as we've matured when we think about food. Part of being naturally thin is waking up and recognizing that you are in charge of your own body, your own mind, and your own life. You make the choices. You are driving, and with this power comes responsibility and a very important recognition that leads me to rule 2:

You can have it all, just not all at once.

This rule is the one to apply when you are faced with a lot of really delicious, fattening, decadent foods. And who isn't faced with them, on a regular basis, living in this country? The good news is that you really can eat anything you want. I've already told you to quit dieting, but just in case you didn't believe me, I'm going to keep saying it. Dieting is *not* helping you; it's hurting you and subtly undermining your own personal power. It also negatively alters your metabolism. I'm serious about this. Diets, by definition, tell you what to eat. Why should anybody else tell you what to eat? What does anybody else know about what you need and desire? It's your body, your taste buds, your preference, *your life.*

But if you are going to call the shots about what you are going to eat, you also have to know what you are doing. You can have the cheeseburger, or the fries, or the strawberry shake. But you can't have them all at once. Hence, rule 2: *You can have it all, just not all at once.*

If your dietary choices have been guided by lust for food and fear of food, then you need this rule, and you need it right now.

Rule 2 actually encapsulates a concept I want you to think very carefully about as you read this chapter. This is something you might not have thought about before. If somebody had told me this years ago, and if I had listened and believed it, I could have saved myself a lot of anxiety. Are you ready? OK, here it is: *you are the only one responsible for what you put into your mouth.*

Obvious? Sure. Revolutionary? Absolutely.

The problem with having so much cheap food available to us is that we tend to *use* it, rather than *eat* it. We use food for entertainment, pleasure, power. We get obsessed with it, and fear it at the same time. Food provides us with plenty of excuses, too. It's not *your* fault that your friends keep wanting you to go out for dinner, or your family wants pizza, or you can't resist those takeout noodles, or you're hungry and the drive-through is *right there.* Or it's PMS or you are dating or you are on vacation or your heart is broken. It's easy to blame the fast-food restaurant, the appealing grocery store display, the dessert cart, girls' night out, your junk-food-junkie friends, your parents, your kids, who leave all that food on their plates, or whoever. Feel free to add your own personal scapegoat to this list. Whatever it is, it's not an excuse. If I could eat healthy on *Martha Stewart: Apprentice,* you can eat healthy during the stressful times in your life.

My point is: it's always somebody else's fault, right? You can't possibly help eating the whole double cheeseburger and the fries, right? *Because they were there.* And how bad does feeling full and bloated feel? Think about whether that feeling outweighs the joy of overeating.

CELEBRITY SECRETS

Years ago, I used to be a personal assistant for Kathy Hilton, and she used to send me to pick up Paris and Nicky at school. I wasn't exactly a babysitter—I was more responsible for running her errands—but sometimes I would take Paris and Nicky ice skating or take them to the Mini Mart for a snack. Paris Hilton is naturally thin, but she never forbids herself any food she wants. If she wants a cheeseburger and fries, she'll order them. If she wants chips or candy, that's what she gets. But she never feels compelled to finish the whole thing. She is a great practitioner of naturally thin strategies, which come to her naturally. If you love decadent foods, Paris Hilton is a good model for how to eat to be naturally thin. I'm not saying you have to practice everything she does, but in this particular aspect of her life, she is definitely a great example.

So quit whining right now about how helpless you are, about how you are a victim because of all that good food around. It's absurd. (Not that I haven't done it too, but I still recognize the absurdity!) Look, you are incredibly lucky to live in a country with so much food, and you have the opportunity to *pick and choose what you want to eat.* Not everybody gets to do this. The beauty of this rule is that you not only gain control of your food choices but get to enjoy, rather than fear, the food in your life. You *can* have it all. You can eat any food you want to eat. No food is forbidden, ever.

But that doesn't mean the rules of the physical universe have been suspended just for your dietary pleasure. If you are going to eat something that has a lot of fat or a lot of calories, or both, you can't *also* eat a lot of other things that have a lot of fat and calories, all at the same time. 💛 *You can have it all, just not all at once.* 💛

Besides, you're not in preschool. Are you trying to make yourself sick? You are an adult, and you don't need pizza *and* ice cream. But pizza *or* ice cream? No problem. Pick what you want, what you really want most, and enjoy it. A little of it. Next time, you can choose something else. Life is about checks and balances, and so is being naturally thin.

Let's look at the implications of this revolutionary rule.

Knowing What You Want

Part of making rule 2 work is learning to recognize what you really want. This isn't always as easy as it sounds, but once you know what you want, eating actually becomes easier than ever before. Isn't everything in life easier when you know what you really want? Relationships, careers, where to live, who to hang around with, what to do with your life, what charities to get involved in—it all makes more sense if you know what you really want. Not what someone else wants. Not what you think you are supposed to want. *What you really want.*

Listening to your food voice is the key to learning what you really want. Do you really want ice cream, or do you just think you want it because everybody else is getting some? Do you really want to eat the leftover chicken fingers and grilled cheese from your child's plate, or would you rather sit down and eat something you will really enjoy?

Understanding and tuning in to your true food desires takes some practice, and some keen listening to the quiet but persistent whisper of your food voice. Don't look for external cues in your environment to help you. You have to tune in to your body and your internal cues, as well as your knowledge from the past about how a food is likely to make you feel.

But right now, you might feel frustrated about how to listen, and how to decide if your thoughts or cravings are based on your food voice or coming out of destructive food noise. There are a lot of ways to do this. Here's what I do:

- If something sounds really good to me—something I know isn't the smartest investment—I try to distract myself. I switch lanes, mentally and physically, and often, I forget all about the craving.
- If I can't stop thinking about it, I probably want it, so I decide to have a small portion. The key is that I *decide* to have it. I'm in control.
- If I can't stop thinking about a decadent food but I know that I saw a picture of it or smelled it or someone else suggested it, I question my first impulse. Maybe it's just convenient, or a habit. Maybe it's just food noise. I spend some time seriously asking myself, Do I *really want it*? Maybe yes, maybe no, but asking yourself is important.

I question my food impulses a lot, just to keep myself in check. When you ask yourself if you *really want* a certain food you are craving, listen. Right away, you'll be stopping yourself from eating automatically, without thinking. Make a decision, consciously and with forethought, and you're already on the right track.

HEAVY HABIT

You want french fries or a banana split right this second? You aren't two years old. Are you going to have a tantrum if you don't get what you want immediately? You may think you want something that you know is not a good investment, but this doesn't mean you have to gratify your every whim. Sometimes, it's worthwhile to decide to indulge in something. But be sure you are doing this with your mature mind in control. Let your food voice, not your inner two-year-old, tell you what you are going to do. Then you'll be able to enjoy your choice without guilt or regret.

If you decide you really want something, then indulge. Otherwise, you will eventually rebel against the unfair restrictions you are putting on yourself, and you'll end up eating twice the calories you would have eaten otherwise. But (here's the key), when you do indulge, really enjoy yourself. When the food becomes even a little less enjoyable—when you've reached the *point of diminishing returns*—then stop.

And if you don't stop? Give yourself a break. Shrug it off. Chalk it up to experience, and *move on*. Now you know even more about your own personal vulnerabilities so you can avoid them more effectively next time. Forgive yourself, and when you have your next meal, balance it. If you ate too much of something sweet, have some protein and vegetables for the next meal. Remember your bank account. When you overspend, you need to rein yourself in for a while. But treat yourself well. Be nice. Nobody deserves to be punished for eating too many cookies.

How Rule 2 Works in Real Life

This rule is particularly useful during those times when you are faced with too many choices. Let's say you are going to a cocktail party. When you arrive, you see a huge array of amazing food—meat trays, cheese trays, dessert trays, vegetable platters, fruit plates, and an open bar. You have to pick your battles. *You can have it all, just not all at once.*

First, do a lap around the table. Look at everything. Feast on it all with your eyes, and pay attention. Maybe that bowl of shrimp doesn't actually look as fresh as you thought at first. Or maybe it looks really amazing. Maybe the cheese is ordinary cheese, or maybe it's your favorite kind. Maybe the desserts look pretty, but on closer examination they don't look all that great—except for those mini cheesecakes. Look at everything and see what really strikes your fancy and what you can admire but can still resist trying.

Now, step back for a minute. Talk to some friends. Have something to drink. When you notice that you really are hungry and ready to eat something, make a plan. Which foods looked best? And how could you balance them? What do you really want, and what can you let go?

Maybe the guacamole looks great, so you have a couple of chips and a healthy scoop of guacamole. Add some salsa or salad or some raw vegetables, to help you fill up on good-investment foods. And what about protein? A little protein will help fill you up and keep you from overeating, so choose the best-looking protein on the table: maybe a slice of turkey or a cube of cheese. But don't go overboard. A few bites should be plenty, and you'll save room for one of those mini cheesecakes. Have some water. Now, do you really need any more than that? You had your favorite things. And you aren't full. And you don't feel guilty. Congratulations. Now forget about the food and go talk to your friends.

This works at home, too. Say you are cooking for your family, and you make a roast chicken. Do you go crazy on the side dishes? Think about what you are doing to yourself and your family when you add mashed potatoes, broccoli, green salad, soup, fruit salad, and a loaf of bread, plus wine or juice and ice cream for dessert. If you fill up on a big green salad and some vegetable soup, you'll have room for only one slice of delicious juicy chicken and maybe a small slice of bread or a small scoop of mashed potatoes (although the broccoli will do more for you than the bread). Balance your choices, but don't pick too many things or you'll wind up eating more than you need. Pick the few best things you want the most, and leave the other dishes for another meal.

Whether you are in a restaurant, out with friends, at someone's house for dinner, or cooking in your own home, this rule can be very powerful. Let it work for you, and use it to nourish your family in a healthy way, too. You can't eliminate food noise completely, but you can definitely turn down the volume and quit letting it control you. Just remember: *you can have it all, just not all at once.*

NATURALLY THIN THOUGHT

When I think about all the food noise I've had to overcome because of the unhealthy lessons I learned growing up, it makes me cringe. If you have kids, one of the most wonderful things you can do for them is to *start them young*. Teach them these rules and bring them up with a healthy attitude to food. Show them how to balance their choices. Show them how much is enough, and don't put so much emphasis on food.

Banish the word *diet* from your house! Kids should never have to hear this four-letter word. My mother was absolutely obsessed with food and dieting, and it took me thirty-five years to undo the damage. Instead, expose your kids to healthy foods like vegetables and fruits from the very beginning, and they won't ever have to unlearn anything. They might even grow up without any food noise at all. Just imagine!

You have greater power than you realize as you bring up your kids. Take off the pressure and bring on the joy of eating. Food isn't love and it isn't an obligation. But it can be an enjoyable way to enhance health. Let it be that for your kids, and you will have done something very good.

Rule 2 Recipes

♡ *You can have it all, just not all at once.* ♡ So pick what you really want, and have it in the best possible way. Is it pasta? Consider the *differential*—would this recipe for whole wheat fusilli with tomato, basil, pine nuts, and smoked mozzarella be just as satisfying as a less nutritious pasta dish? If so, go for this one. It tastes great, it's filling, and it's full of protein, fiber, and vitamins, but it isn't nearly as high in fat and calories as something like lasagna or spaghetti with meat sauce.

Or maybe you are in the mood for dessert. You can indulge if you want to, but maybe my faux cheesecake recipe would be just as good. Give it a try. It might become one of your new favorite foods.

Whole Wheat Fusilli with Tomato, Basil, Pine Nuts, and Smoked Mozzarella

This delicious recipe makes an excellent dinner, but you can also make it ahead (or double it) and have the leftovers for lunch the next day. You can substitute brown rice pasta for the whole wheat pasta if you avoid gluten, or use white pasta—although white pasta is not as good for you and tends to stimulate the appetite, so go easy on it. As for the cheese, you can leave out the smoked mozzarella and instead use ricotta, feta, or shredded Parmesan. You don't need very much of these high-flavor cheeses to get a satisfying cheese experience, but don't leave it out. The protein balances the carbs. Serve with a salad.

Serves 2 (You can halve or double the recipe if that works better for you.)

½ cup whole wheat fusilli

2 teaspoons olive oil

2 to 3 cloves of garlic, smashed, peeled, and minced (whack the cloves with the side of a large knife for easier peeling)

4 Roma tomatoes, chopped

Salt and pepper, to taste

½ cup fresh shredded basil plus 2 tablespoons for garnish

1 tablespoon toasted pine nuts (see page 29 for toasting directions)

2 ounces smoked mozzarella, shredded

1. Cook the pasta according to package directions, until firm but tender (al dente).

2. While the pasta is cooking, heat the olive oil in a nonstick skillet. Sauté the garlic in the oil until golden but not brown. Add the tomatoes, salt, and pepper. Simmer until the pasta is done cooking.

3. Remove the pasta from the water with a slotted spoon and add it to the sauce. Add about ¼ cup of the pasta cooking water as you go. This helps thicken the sauce.

4. Stir in the ½ cup shredded basil, pine nuts, and mozzarella. Stir to combine. Remove to two plates and garnish with more shredded basil. Serve hot.

Bethenny's Faux Cheesecake

This recipe is quick and easy but so good that it can curb the most raging sweet tooth. You can be creative with this recipe, adding dark chocolate chips, fruit, or a different kind of nut. Customize this faux cheesecake for your craving, and savor every bite.

Serves 1 (You can double it for two people if you want to serve it for dessert.)

½ cup whipped cottage cheese (Friendship makes a great one) or low-fat ricotta cheese

½ teaspoon vanilla or almond extract (or lemon, pistachio)

1 tablespoon dark chocolate chips *or* slivered almonds or anything else that goes with the flavor

1 teaspoon honey or maple syrup

Combine all the ingredients in a small bowl or ramekin. Eat immediately, or cover and chill.

Chapter 3

TASTE EVERYTHING, EAT NOTHING

Now that you are balancing your diet every day, and are working to integrate the concept of having anything you want, just not all at once, you are ready for rule 3. This is one of the most misunderstood rules, but also one of the most powerful, and one of my personal favorites. People sometimes overreact to the sound of it, but that's just because they don't fully understand its meaning. Rule 3 is actually simple:

Taste everything, eat nothing.

Now settle down, I don't really mean that you can't eat anything. That's what people think when they hear this rule: they think I'm saying that you can never eat a whole portion of anything again. Of course I'm not saying this. You will eat plenty of full portions of things. But you don't always need to do it. In fact, *not* doing it much of the time can be a powerful tool for becoming naturally thin, and that's what this rule is all about.

At its heart, this rule helps you to taste little bits of all the delicious foods you want, without eating too much of any one thing. Sometimes, you will follow rule 2 (*You can have it all, just not all at once*), and choose to have one or two really good things. At other times, when there are so many amazing choices that you can't limit yourself, you can have little tastes of a lot of different things. You can feel that you really have participated in life and in all the delicious foods a situation has to offer, without overdoing it. This dynamic rule 3 will be the key to getting through some of life's trickier situations, in which overeating is too easy: cocktail parties, tailgate parties, dinner parties, Super Bowl parties full of fried food, upscale restaurants, fast-food restaurants, traveling, convenience stores, and even home-cooked meals. On Thanksgiving, when you risk gorging and falling asleep for hours, rule 3 is crucial. This rule will give you the power to face these situations without fear. You'll be able to taste all the best foods you love, while still eating to be naturally thin.

Mangia Poco Ma Bene

I love the Italian saying *Mangia poco ma bene*. It means "Eat little, but well." It means quality versus quantity. It's not exactly the same as *Taste everything, eat nothing,* but it has the same sentiment behind it: the best way to eat is to eat little bits of really great food. I mention it here because I first came up with this rule when I was in Italy, where people truly understand how to eat this way.

As far as I can see, here's what most people in America actually do: eat everything and taste nothing. We stuff ourselves while staring at television, answering e-mails, or driving, and we hardly taste what we eat, let alone remember eating it. How else do you explain all the sub-par fake food we are always stuffing into our faces?

But the Italians don't live that way. They eat what they want to eat—some of everything—but they never eat very much of it, and it is always good, fresh, real food. *Sample.* That's the key. Italy is where I learned to ♡ *taste everything, eat nothing.* ♡ If the idea of your diet as a bank account is the soul of this book, rule 3 is the heart.

Here's an example of how I used this rule in Italy. I started each morning with a cappuccino, with real full-fat milk, the way the Italians drink it. They don't drink "skinny lattes." Nor was I going to be the annoying person I was in the past, asking for skim milk and sugar-free sweetener. Italians don't really use artificial sweetener: they use real sugar.

With my cappuccino, I would eat a small amount of fruit with a small pastry, or a small piece of bread with cheese. The key here is *small.* This way, I could have the cappuccino, the fruit, and the pastry—a few bites or sips of each. I didn't feel compelled to actually finish any of it, because the key here was to *taste* it all.

For lunch or dinner, I would have some pasta, but at only one of those meals, and only a small order. I rarely finished it all. I would always combine the pasta with something light and filling (always go for volume when filling up), like grilled vegetables or salad. I also included a little protein. For the other main meal, I focused more on protein, such as lean meat, poultry, or fish (because I remembered that my diet is a bank account).

I wasn't going to miss out on the gelato, either—this is one of Italy's most wonderful culinary treasures, in my opinion. Every day, I would have a small gelato in the afternoon, *or* a few bites of dessert after dinner. But I never had both. The same goes for wine, another Italian specialty. I try to limit myself to two drinks per day, either wine or clear liquor. In Italy, either I would choose the meal best accompanied by wine, or I would split my allowance and have one glass with lunch and one glass with dinner. OK, sometimes I had three. I was on vacation!

Because I planned my investments this way, I never felt that I missed out on anything. When I got back from Italy, my jeans fit exactly the way they did before I left, and I realized that I had been eating the way humans are supposed to eat—tasting little bits of the very best foods, the foods I wanted the most. I had been eating to be naturally thin—without deprivation, without dieting. I never looked back. Now, I practice this way of eating all the time.

You are going to love the way this rule helps you to stop fearing food. No food is fattening, in a small quantity. Weight is a simple equation of calories in, calories out. A giant bowl of healthy whole-wheat pasta with no oil, topped with grilled vegetables, has more calories than a few bites of, for example, cheesy lasagna or spaghetti with meatballs. You have to decide how to invest and what is more important. I would rather sample a little of everything, so I don't miss out on anything. Variety is the spice of life.

Spoil Your Appetite

Spoiling your appetite is, in a way, its own rule, although it is closely linked with rule 3 because it makes rule 3 possible. If you are ravenous, you're going to have a hard time just tasting something great. But if you have spoiled your appetite? No problem.

Although a lot of people overeat because they don't pay attention to when they have had enough, they usually *start* overeating because of excessive hunger. When you are too hungry, it's much harder to make rational choices about what foods would be best to eat. And portion control? Forget about it. If you're starving, you're going to pile it on. We've all been there. It's one of the biggest reasons why people binge.

This concept is directly related to ♡ *taste everything, eat nothing* ♡ because if you are starving, you are not going to be able to just taste. You are going to eat the whole thing, and more. But it's your life, your body, and your food choices, so it's up to you to make sure you never get to the point where you are starving and can't make those smart decisions. The best way I know to do that is to spoil your appetite.

To do this the right way, however, you have to plan ahead. When you know you are going to an event that will offer a lot of opportunities for overeating (like a party with a buffet table or a restaurant with really great desserts), and you know it's going to be a ♡ *taste*

CELEBRITY SECRETS

I met Charles Barclay at a spa in California where celebrities pay $3,000 to starve and hike twelve to fifteen miles per day. Charles and I became great friends while we were there. I remember when we were on a sixteen-mile hike together. While I was eating the single apple we were allowed to eat for breakfast, he turned to me and said, "I'll carry you an extra mile for one of them apple slices." He's beyond hilarious and we're still friends, but I always remember that feeling—being so hungry that you just can't stand it. You'll do anything. You'll *eat* anything. Sure, Charles is in great shape, and he uses these boot camps for cleansing. But he knows that he can't always live like that. Nobody can. People go for one week a year and spend the next fifty-one weeks waiting until they go back to be "good" again. That explains why I only went once. To me, it makes a whole lot more sense (and costs a whole lot less money) to eat right every day. Then you never need to go to such extremes.

everything, eat nothing scenario, the worst thing you can do is to starve yourself all day because you think that starving will allow you to eat more. Do just the opposite. Eat a simple, sensible breakfast; have a healthy, light lunch (see some suggestions at the end of this chapter); and then, right before you go to the party, have a healthy snack. You might be surprised to learn that a packaged veggie burger with a slice of soy cheese on one slice of whole-grain toast has less than 250 calories. That's an amazing investment, because you'll feel as if you had a full meal, and you won't overeat later. You'll *taste everything, eat nothing* with no problem.

People are so afraid to do this! They think that eating before a party will add way too many calories. Trust me—it's not true. The calories you will save by eating sensibly and having a healthful snack before you are faced with temptation will more than make up for the calories you spend. This is a good investment strategy for eating.

Don't choose just any snack when you are spoiling your appetite before a big event. Choose something nourishing and filling. Don't make this a day for decadent snacks like chocolate or ice cream, since you are balancing your diet like a bank account and you know you will have more decadent choices at the party or restaurant.

NATURALLY THIN THOUGHT

Great snack options include a slice of whole-grain bread with nut butter or hummus; a small handful of nuts; edamame; a slice of turkey and a slice of Swiss cheese; low-fat yogurt with a few berries and some nuts mixed in, or some pureed vegetable soup or gazpacho.

Spoiling your appetite with smart snacking is a good investment in your immediate and long-term future. You'll be able to enjoy just a few tastes of the very best things, and then you'll go home respecting yourself, feeling powerful and in control of your own behavior. And that's a much better feeling than hating yourself because you ate too much.

But you don't need a big event to spoil your appetite. You can do it every day. Have you ever skipped lunch and then gone overboard for dinner because you were starving? Or have you ever felt virtuous eating nothing but a small salad for dinner, than gone wild with hunger late at night and finished off a whole bag of chips? That's because you forgot to spoil your appetite.

Ordering in a Restaurant

Restaurants are great places to practice rule 3. When I go to a restaurant, I basically ignore the entrée list because to me, all the other things—the soups, salads, side dishes, and appetizers—are more interesting and offer more opportunities for tasting a lot of amazing things in small portions. I talk more about eating in restaurants in the second part of this book, but I want you to have the tools you need now, so let's talk about how to use rule 3 the very next time you go out to eat.

When I go to a restaurant, the first thing I do is read the menu and make a plan. I usually zero in on the appetizers and sides. I love ordering appetizers and sides because they allow me to taste a lot of great foods and balance my meal so I'm not getting too much of any one thing. Usually, I choose two appetizers or an appetizer and a side dish. One of the first plates is usually something like salad or a bowl of soup, something with a lot of vegetables that will fill me up with high volume and not too much fat or too many calories.

The second appetizer or side is usually something a little more decadent, like a small plate of pasta, a crab cake, or an antipasto platter with a small selection of high-quality cheeses and meats. This is common sense. Don't get really decadent appetizers, like fried calamari and french fries. Your body doesn't want them, and you are striving for balance. Balance the fried calamari with the salad. Balance the fried crab cake with the vegetables. Listen to your food voice. Indulge with one small plate, and nourish your body with the other.

That leaves me room to try other things, too—a few bites of a friend's steak or dessert or a few sips of an after-dinner drink, or whatever I really want. I might also have my trademark SkinnyGirl Margarita™ for a small amount of intense flavor (see the recipe at the end of this chapter). After it's all over, you can bet I'll feel satisfied. I tried everything I wanted.

NATURALLY THIN THOUGHT

Tasting menus can be a fun way to try lots of different things, but even tasting menus can sometimes give you portions that are too large. Literally just taste, and you'll get plenty of food. You want to eat not until you feel full but just until you feel satisfied.

Switching Lanes

Another problem some people face when they try to practice rule 3, *taste everything, eat nothing,* is that they enjoy the taste of something so much that it overrides their sense of hunger or satiety and they just keep eating. This is when I like to practice a strategy I call *switching lanes.*

Switching lanes means that when you eat a little of something you really love, instead of allowing yourself to keep going simply because of the pleasurable taste, you make yourself stop after a few bites, and move to a different taste. This jolts your taste buds out of their mindless reverie, so you don't overdo it. The new food might not necessarily be a good investment food, but the point is that it stops the momentum.

I use this strategy all the time. Sometimes it works. Sometimes it doesn't. But it almost always tells me whether my cravings are genuine, or based on some other, nonfood emotion.

Let me give you an example. Recently, I had a serious craving for a cupcake—I think I would have exploded if I didn't have an iced cupcake. So, following my own advice, I had a small one, but it was so good that I felt I just had to have another. Well, we all know where that can lead. So instead of having another, I switched lanes. I changed what I was eating to break the cycle of that taste. I had a small piece of real dark chocolate with almonds (for the protein to control blood sugar), took a deep breath—and I was fine. My cupcake craving was gone.

But that's not always the way it works. A few weeks ago, a friend and I ordered Chinese takeout. I had mu shu chicken, and it tasted really good, so I ate half. This seemed like a sensible portion, but when I got to the end of it, I wanted to keep eating. But did I want more just because it was there and it tasted so good, or was I really still hungry? I wasn't sure, but I was pretty sure I'd had enough food, so I switched lanes. I ate a small scoop of Ben & Jerry's low-fat ice cream, thinking I would be done with it.

But I wasn't done with it. I kept thinking about that mu shu pork until I realized that I really, genuinely wanted to eat the rest of it. Switching lanes wasn't going to change that. I finished it. However, the strategy did clarify to me that my desire for more mu shu pork wasn't based in mindless eating. I really did want it, so I had it. It was a learning experience. I'm human, and so are you.

When you ♡ *taste everything, eat nothing,* ♡ what you are actually doing is switching lanes throughout the meal. A few bites of this, then a few bites of that, then a few bites of something else. You keep switching lanes so you never go off on a tear. It's exactly what allows you to enjoy all your favorite foods.

And when it doesn't work? You are learning the difference between your food noise and your food voice, that's all.

Rule 3 Recipes

When you ♡ *taste everything, eat nothing,* ♡ it's important to taste only the very best foods, or make the foods you taste as healthy as possible without compromising taste. Here are two of my favorite high-taste, low-impact recipes. These are delicious, decadent, but, healthy comfort foods. Enjoy, but don't overindulge. Taste!

Zesty, Cheesy, Healthy Mac and Cheese

This recipe is amazing—the best macaroni and cheese you've ever had, with great flavor but a fraction of the fat and calories the old fashioned kind has. This is true comfort food. Just remember to *taste* it and don't overdo it.

Serves 4 (not 1!)

12 ounces whole wheat mini pasta shells (these hold the cheese better than elbows)

1 cup soymilk

1 cup freshly shredded Parmesan cheese (must be Parmigiano-Reggiano—the real stuff)

1 cup reduced-fat sharp cheddar cheese, shredded

1 cup frozen butternut squash thawed

1 teaspoon salt, plus more if needed

1 teaspoon dry mustard

½ teaspoon pepper, plus more if needed

½ teaspoon Worcestershire sauce

½ teaspoon chili powder, or a few dashes of Tabasco sauce

2 tablespoons whole wheat bread crumbs

2 tablespoons reduced-fat Monterey jack cheese, shredded

1. Boil the pasta shells in salted water until slightly firm, or according to the package directions. Preheat the oven to 350°F.

2. In another saucepan, combine soymilk, Parmesan, cheddar, and butternut squash over medium heat until melted and combined. Turn off heat. Add salt, mustard, pepper, Worcestershire, and chili powder or Tabasco.

3. Drain pasta (don't rinse) and combine with cheese sauce in another bowl. Taste and add additional salt and pepper as needed.

4. Place in a shallow baking dish sprayed with nonstick cooking spray, sprinkle with breadcrumbs and Monterey jack cheese, and bake for 15 to 20 minutes, or until slightly browned.

"Out of this World" Stuffing

This stuffing really is out of this world. It provides you with all the comforting goodness of bread stuffing with just a fraction of the calories and fat traditional stuffing has. This recipe has a lot of ingredients, but the actual process is easy.

Serves 6 to 8

1 large onion, chopped

3 stalks of celery, finely chopped

1 tablespoon olive oil

½ teaspoon salt, plus more as needed

½ teaspoon pepper, plus more as needed

1 or 2 cloves fresh garlic, minced

4 sprigs sage, finely chopped

Leaves from 6 to 8 sprigs of thyme, finely chopped

½ pound turkey sausage (It comes in different flavors, so choose your favorite.
 I recommend the fennel flavor.)

Splash of good dry white wine

1 teaspoon butter

1 pound fresh mushrooms, sliced (whatever kind you like, or try an assortment)

½ cup dried morels, coarsely chopped and soaked in water until soft

½ loaf of 9-grain or multi-grain bread, toasted and chopped

½ to 1 cup chicken stock, mushroom broth, white wine, or other flavored liquid, if
 necessary

1 egg, beaten

Cooking spray

1. Preheat the oven to 350°F. Sauté the onion and celery in the oil, in a nonstick pan. Add the salt, pepper, garlic, sage, and thyme.

2. Take the sausage out of its casing (if it is in a casing) and break it into small pieces. Add to the pan and sauté until browned. Add the wine and butter. Stir in the mushrooms, morels, and morel soaking water.

3. Put the bread crumbs in a large bowl. Pour the sausage mixture over the top and toss to coat. If the mixture seems dry, add the chicken stock, mushroom broth, wine, or other flavored liquid. Add more salt and pepper, to taste. Stir in the beaten egg and mix it all together. Put it into a large baking pan sprayed with cooking spray.

4. Bake for 25 to 30 minutes, then turn the oven to broil. Broil for five minutes to make the top crunchy—but watch it closely to be sure it doesn't burn.

Chapter 4

PAY ATTENTION

When you barrel through the food on your plate as if you are in a race to see who can finish first, do you really taste what you are eating? Did your body even register that it had a meal? Is this any way to be naturally thin?

No, no, and no. Look, I know you're busy, stressed, overworked, all of that. So am I. You are probably keeping a million balls in the air, but that is all the more reason to follow rule 4:

Pay attention.

It's so easy to eat mindlessly without paying attention to what foods we choose, or to how they taste. But to eat consciously changes all that. It makes food an event, and worth the calories. It also helps you become choosier about what you eat. And it helps you eat less.

You would think it would be common sense to pay attention when you do something as important to your health as eat, but most people take eating for granted. We stuff our faces while we watch television, work, drive, or talk on the phone. Who has time to do only one thing at a time? I know I'm usually doing about seven things at once and running around like a crazy woman at the same time, trying to get from one appointment to the next.

But here's the truth: No matter how busy you are, no matter where you have to go next, and no matter how much is going through your brain at any given moment, you can take three minutes to stop, take a breath, and give some thought and attention to what you are eating to nourish yourself. The food you eat gives you the energy you need to keep up your crazy schedule and keep all those balls in the air at the same time. Doesn't it deserve a little respect?

If you are already practicing the first three rules, you are moving toward more conscious eating. Every time you consciously balance your food choices like a bank account (rule 1), consciously choose one thing over another with the realization that you can have it all but not all at once (rule 2), or consciously taste instead of eating (rule 3), you are paying attention (rule 4).

Rule 4 covers much more than the aspects of conscious eating inherent in the first three rules. Eating consciously is an experience in and of itself, and involves a number of techniques you can practice in the same way you might practice yoga, the guitar, or French pronunciation. Eating consciously can become almost a meditation on sensory pleasure. It's also a key to becoming naturally thin.

Eating Consciously 101

When you first start trying to pay attention while you eat, you may find it difficult, especially if you aren't in the habit. In a way, it's comforting to eat mindlessly. You don't have to think about your choices or take responsibility for your actions. Oops—the bag of cookies is empty? Oh, well! You missed the experience, but you don't have to feel guilty if you barely remember eating those cookies. Or do you?

If you ♡ *pay attention* ♡ to your food, you will discover a whole new world of pleasurable sensation that far exceeds the comfort of mindless eating. Don't graze your way mindlessly through life. Make it count. Here are some tips for learning how to eat more consciously:

- **Tune in to your food preparation, no matter how simple.** Appreciate the process, whether you are cooking a fancy meal or scooping ice cream. If you make half a turkey sandwich with Swiss cheese on whole-wheat bread, pay attention to what you are doing and make what you are making special.
- **Taste your food.** This is very important. *If you eat food and you don't pay attention, you'll feel as though you didn't eat.* Then you won't be satisfied. You'll want to eat more. It's a vicious circle, and you need to stop this bad habit now. It takes two seconds to shift your attention to what you are doing and taste what you are eating. Then, the food will register as an experience and it will stick with you.
- **Chew your food slowly and well.** You can taste your food better if you chew it all the way, and you'll digest it better, too. This is a big reason why I take longer to eat than most of my friends, and the result is that I eat less.
- **Notice when other people aren't paying attention.** Soon you will become aware of how people eat mindlessly while cooking, nibble through a whole box of crackers, or pick food off other people's plates. I can't stand seeing people picking at food while they cook (or while *I* cook!). It's not pretty, and it's certainly not what naturally thin people do.
- **Be a bit of a food snob.** If you really ♡ *pay attention* ♡ to your food, you'll start noticing when it doesn't look appealing or doesn't taste very good. Then you'll be in a position to turn down food that doesn't meet your standards.
- **Quit multitasking.** If somebody told me to quit multitasking, I would laugh. My life wouldn't work if I didn't do a million things at once. But we don't have to carry that stress-inducing way of life into mealtimes. When we do, not only do we fail to di-

NATURALLY THIN THOUGHT

I don't mean for you to go overboard or get obsessive about eating consciously. It's unrealistic every time you need to eat something to expect yourself to sit down for an hour and focus so intensely on every bite that you miss what's going on around you. That not only would make meals huge time-consuming events, but would defeat the whole purpose of enjoying all the other aspects of eating, including socializing and ambience. However, even if your meal or snack lasts just two minutes, you can still focus on what you are doing. You should at least *remember* eating!

gest our food as well or enjoy it as much, but we tend to eat more of it. So, I want you to make a new policy for yourself: don't eat while doing something else. I know this isn't always possible, but it's a good goal. Sometimes, you have no other choice but to grab something quick in the car or eat while you are finishing up a job on the computer. If you must, at least be mindful and aware while you are doing it. If you have to eat an energy bar in the car, pay attention, take little bites, and taste it.

- **Think like an Italian.** In Europe, eating is an event. Food seems to matter more to Europeans, and I would say that food is more important to the Italians than work or even money. If savoring and treasuring really high-quality food were actually important to you, don't you think you would be a bit healthier? But at the same time, Europeans aren't nearly as obsessed with food as we are in America. How do they pull that off? Instead of obsessing over food, they respect it by giving it their full attention. Although Europe is getting more Americanized, in general, the Europeans would be horrified by the idea of eating in front of the television set or while driving. In fact, a lot of European cars don't even have drink holders. Many Europeans wouldn't think of bringing a massive beverage from a convenience store into their cars. When you eat, you

> **HEAVY HABIT**
>
> Turn off the television! Studies have proved that when you eat while watching television, you eat a lot more than you would if you were just eating without doing anything else. It's amazing how much more you will eat when distracted by other things, too. If you tend to eat lunch at your desk while working or in the car while driving, you'll discover that quitting this habit really will help you eat less and feel calmer. I'm not saying that you have to act like a member of the royal family and demand that all activity cease around you because you want to eat a sandwich. But why shouldn't you sit down and eat in a calm, civilized manner? Eat something, *then* watch your favorite show.

eat. When you drive, you drive. When you watch television, you watch television. When you work, you work. Try it.

- **Take a seat.** I can tell you to eat consciously all day, but I know perfectly well that it's hard to do if you are in the habit of distracted eating. One easy, powerful strategy for helping yourself remember to pay attention is *never eat while standing up*. Or, to put this in more positive terms, *always sit down to eat*. When you eat while standing up, whether you are cooking, snacking, or just picking at food, you won't feel satisfied, because you aren't really thinking about eating. You get the feeling the food you eat while standing up doesn't really count. But believe me, it counts. So if you consciously decide to eat something, put it on a plate, sit down, and pay attention to it.

- **Slow down.** It's easy to feel pressure to eat quickly. We have a schedule, or the people we are eating with are already done. But you don't have to think or eat like that. I no longer feel pressure to rush through a meal. I refuse. I believe it is more civilized to enjoy a meal calmly. Focus on the conversation, the atmosphere, and what you are eating. Don't gobble uncontrollably. I often eat with people who finish in half the time it

---

HEAVY HABIT

I have a friend who likes to stand over me and graze in the kitchen while I cook. Not only is this annoying to me, but he has no idea how many calories he consumes while casually noshing on what is about to become dinner. This is especially easy to do during the holidays, when there is so much good food around all the time. But remember this: if you taste only what you need to taste to make sure the dishes you are cooking taste good, but don't eat until you are ready to make yourself a plate and sit down to your meal, you will save hundreds of unnecessary calories. Cooking is no excuse to stuff your face before dinner even starts. As a chef, I know how important it is to taste the food as I cook, to be sure it's right, but I consider that part of my dinner and I balance it out when I sit down. I don't mindlessly snack while cooking because if I did, I wouldn't have any room left in my account for an actual meal—and to me, that wouldn't be worth the price.

---

takes me, and ten minutes later, they cannot believe how over-whelmingly full they are. You should never feel uncomfortably full. Feel satisfied. There will always be another meal.

- **Pause between bites.** I also think it's important to pause after every bite or two. Take a breath, and do a quick mental check. Am I full yet? Have I reached the *point of diminishing returns*? (Reminder: that is the point where the food isn't quite as good as it was when you first started eating it.) If you are full, or you've reached the point of maximum enjoyment and it's only going to get less pleasurable, stop. This pause will give you the chance to do so. If you eat too quickly, your food will be gone before you even feel as if you've started eating.

- **Calm yourself.** One reason some of us have such a hard time eating consciously is that we aren't calm. When you are in an agitated, excited, or really busy state of mind, it's extremely hard to eat consciously. But stop, breathe, calm yourself, and you'll suddenly see how easy and pleasurable it is to pay attention. By the same token, if you are feeling really anxious or upset about something, it's usually a good idea *not* to eat. Eating when you aren't calm not only contributes to the habit of trying to drown out emotions with food but also tends to result in overeating without any pleasure. All you feel is guilty. So wait to eat until you've calmed down. Stretch, breathe, do a little yoga—do anything to quiet your food noise before you dig in.

- **Make food special.** In a restaurant or at a spa, you pay to have your food made special. It looks beautiful and is fun to eat. So why shouldn't you do that for yourself at home? If your food is really worth it, you'll be more likely to pay attention and let eating become an experience. Consider the humble cheese sandwich. You can throw a slice of cheese onto a piece of bread and eat it, and that will do if you are starving. But what if you toasted a really high-quality piece of whole-grain bread, spread it with Dijon mustard, gently melted a slice of low-fat cheese on it, added a fresh slice of bright red tomato, and seasoned it with a little salt and pepper? This is a snack that will taste so much more interesting and special, with hardly any more effort. You might not really notice the taste of the plain cheese on the plain bread, but when you make the food special, that food will get your attention and you'll eat more consciously. To make a salad, don't just grab some iceberg lettuce out of a bag. Choose fresh crisp greens, then top them with a sprinkle of nuts or shaved Parmesan, or a few crumbles of feta cheese. Add fresh or dried herbs, lemon zest, and just a splash of your favorite dressing. Don't just pour milk over cereal in a mug for breakfast. Sprinkle almonds and raisins on your cereal, then add milk and a drizzle of maple syrup, for a hearty breakfast treat. Taking a little extra time to make your meal special will help you to feel so much more satisfied and content with your food.

When it comes to food (or anything else), I always say, "Good enough just isn't." As with everything in life, make your food as special as possible. The rewards are endless. It really takes only a few extra minutes, so please don't use "I don't have time" as an excuse. Your health is more important than anything else in the world, and eating consciously will do amazing things for your life.

NATURALLY THIN THOUGHT

Another good way to make your food special is to make sure it is colorful. This is one of the most important concepts for health, and it is so simple that you can take this piece of advice with you anywhere. If a food has a bright color that occurs naturally, then it is probably very good for you. Blueberries (all berries), pumpkins, pomegranates, sweet potatoes, broccoli, carrots, asparagus, kale, collard greens, beets, etc., are all healthful and inviting because of their beautiful, vibrant color. Always opt for the brightest color. Although cauliflower is a good high-volume, high-fiber food, if given the option I'd sooner have broccoli because of its bright color. Color makes food both beautiful and nutritious.

Watch What You Watch

Before I finish this chapter, I have to say something in particular about the media. The power of a television commercial, a billboard, or a sign outside a restaurant is amazing. Advertisers know what they are doing, but that doesn't mean you have to become the next victim.

If I see some food on television that looks really good, I'll start craving it, even if I don't really want it. You might notice that when the Super Bowl comes around, or the holiday season starts, you'll see an extra onslaught of food commercials. Just seeing ads showing baby back ribs, cheeseburgers, roasted turkeys, or sugar cookies can make you want them. If you are susceptible to that kind of appeal (and most of us are), don't give in. Change the channel. There is no reason to sit there, tempting fate and testing yourself beyond endurance.

Along those same lines, don't let yourself get overly obsessed with food. I'm a chef and I love food, but I don't talk about it constantly. I have a lot of other things in my life to focus on. Talking about and thinking about food constantly can result in eating more than you really need or even want, just because food is on the brain.

Are you sitting there watching cooking shows all evening? Well, stop it. Why are you doing that to yourself? There isn't anything wrong with enjoying great food, but save those food thoughts and reveries for when you are really hungry and want to cook or eat something. If you want to find some good, healthy recipes on the Internet or get some cooking tips from a famous television chef, fine. Just be aware of what you are doing, and the effect it can have. The world is bombarding us with images of food to trick us into eating when we don't really want or need to eat. To ♡ *pay attention* ♡ means more than just eating consciously. It means dealing with food propaganda consciously, too. Remember—you are the one in control of your own mind, body, and choices. ♡ *Pay attention,* ♡ and you'll make better decisions.

Rule 4 Recipes

It's quick and easy to make food special, to help yourself eat more consciously and with greater pleasure. You don't have to be a gourmet cook. These recipes are quick to make at home, and they are full of color, flavor, and good nutrition.

Arugula Salad

Anybody can open a bag of greens and pour dressing on it. That's not special. Try this simple salad instead. It's an *event*. You can find bresaola (thinly sliced air-dried beef) at gourmet or higher-end food stores, either in packages or from the deli.

Serves 4

8 cups arugula, well washed
Salt and pepper, to taste
4 ounces fresh Parmesan

3 tablespoons toasted pine nuts (see page 29 for toasting directions)

Juice of 1 lemon, freshly squeezed

¼ cup extra-virgin olive oil

1 tablespoon truffle oil (optional)

4 to 8 ounces bresaola (optional)

1. Arrange the arugula on a platter. Season with salt and pepper.

2. Using a vegetable peeler, shave the fresh Parmigiano on top of the arugula. Sprinkle with the pine nuts.

3. Drizzle the salad with lemon juice, then olive oil, then truffle oil, if you are using it. You don't need much oil on this salad, because arugula has such high flavor.

4. If you are using the bresaola, arrange the slices around the edges of the platter.

Vegetable Tower

You can order fancy versions of this easy dish in a restaurant, but make it at home to impress guests or just to impress yourself. You'll be surprised how easy it is, especially if you use leftover vegetables that are already cooked.

Serves 1 or 2 (depending on how hungry you are; it's also easy to double or triple)

Cooking spray

2 whole portobello mushrooms about 3–4 inches in diameter, marinated in your favorite low-fat Balsamic vinaigrette and roasted. (While roasting or grilling, weight them down with a heavy pan so they flatten out and release more moisture.)

Salt and pepper, to taste

½ cup fresh spinach, well washed, sautéed with olive oil and garlic

2 sliced sun-dried tomatoes in water, drained

2 ounces feta or mozzarella cheese

1 tablespoon store-bought pesto

1 tablespoon pine nuts

Preheat the oven to 400°F. Spray a baking sheet with cooking spray. Place the two mushroom caps on the baking sheet. Season with salt and pepper. Carefully layer each with half the spinach, tomatoes, and cheese. Bake for about 15 minutes, or until the cheese is melted. Carefully remove to a plate. Drizzle with pesto and sprinkle with pine nuts.

Chapter 5

DOWNSIZE NOW!

What's with that mountain of pasta on your plate? Are you sharing it with five people? What's with the vat of fries? You know the term *supersize*, but I certainly hope that you aren't using that word at the drive-through (hopefully you rarely do go through the drive-through!). In fact, I hope the very thought makes you cringe. If you want to be naturally thin, supersize should not even be on your radar. Instead, let *downsize* be your mantra. That brings us to rule 5.

Downsizing is simple. It means eating smaller portions. Our ideas about portions have become so out of control that in many restaurants, a single entrée could easily feed four people. I don't know who first thought that gigantic platters of pasta, three-pound steaks, or burritos the size of your head were a good idea or even remotely appropriate to serve to one person, much less appealing in any way. I think they're gross, frankly. Huge mountains of food? They're just slovenly, and a poor presentation, not to mention a clear factor in obesity.

I mean this not in a condescending way but just as an exercise: Look around at the waistlines of the people who are eating those huge portions. You can see a direct correlation. Who's in line at the buffet? Is it an accident that the people looking to get the most food for their money are the largest? Food doesn't just fall onto your body and make you fat; you are the one who makes the decision to eat it—and eat more and more and more of it. People think they are getting a better value if they eat more, but as I've said before, eating more and getting fatter and fatter often result in spending more and more money on diets. It's completely illogical to do this. The answer?

♡ Downsize now! ♡

Clearly, America's idea of a portion is out of whack. It's time to separate yourself from all that ridiculous excess. I know we are supposedly living in a land of plenty, but that's no reason to have a body of plenty. Wouldn't you rather have energy, have vitality, and be naturally thin?

CELEBRITY SECRETS

Being a chef, I get the opportunity to meet a lot of other chefs, and they are wonderful advocates of the concept ♡ *downsize now!* ♡ because they are choosy: they use the very best ingredients, and they savor every bite. Rocco DiSpirito is a great example of a chef who makes amazing food that tastes rich and decadent, but serves it in reasonably sized, beautifully crafted portions. Plus, he's incredibly fit. Bobby Flay is another example. His wife, Stephanie March, says because she lives with a chef, she thoroughly understands the ten rules—they describe how people are *supposed* to eat. Enjoy food, eat what you want to eat, but choose real food and don't eat huge amounts. Food should be savored, tasted, and enjoyed, not gorged on. Chefs know this, and now you know it, too.

Downsizing is not deprivation. Actually, it's the opposite. What would make you feel more deprived: a mountain of steamed vegetables and nothing else, or a couple of bites of delicious juicy steak, a small but vibrantly fresh salad, a few pieces of steamy roasted potato, and three bites of moist, delectable chocolate cake?

Downsizing allows you to eat *anything you want,* and that is incredibly freeing. You'll never feel left out or unable to participate. You'll never be shackled by limitations. If your portion is small, you can eat absolutely anything that really sounds good to you. Sometimes just knowing that you are "allowed" to nibble on a few french fries prevents you from overeating. Overeating is often a product of feeling deprived. You deprive and deprive yourself all day. Then you lose control and go crazy, eating everything in sight.

But what if you were never deprived of any food you wanted? Why would you ever bother to go crazy and overeat? Since I stopped depriving myself of the foods I wanted, and instead allowed myself a few perfect bites, I've lost the urge to binge. It just doesn't happen anymore.

But life in twenty-first-century America makes downsizing a challenge, so in this chapter, I'm going to give you some tools to help you downsize in a supersizing world.

Now Means Now

Rule 5, ♡*downsize now!,*♡ means just what it says. Downsize *now.* Not tomorrow. There is no tomorrow. Not after you finish this chapter. Not next week. Not after you've had a huge snack to prepare yourself. *Now.* There is absolutely no reason to wait any longer. There is never any reason to eat a huge oversized portion of anything. There is never any reason to stuff yourself until you feel sick. Remember the *point of diminishing returns.* When the food starts tasting less exciting, stop. That's a portion.

Every time you choose something to eat, you have an opportunity to downsize. But downsizing is a process of conscientious negotiation. If you usually have two pieces of toast for breakfast, would you be perfectly happy and satisfied with just one? What are they, bookends? Why does everybody always think that food has to come in twos? Two fried eggs, two slices of bacon, two pieces of toast. Who says you can't eat one fried egg, one slice of bacon, and one slice of toast?

Are you having two out of habit? If you are having two pieces of toast because one just does not satisfy you and you need two pieces to feel that you've had enough breakfast, then have two pieces. But if one piece with some protein like peanut butter or a piece of cheese and a piece of fresh fruit fills you up, then this downsized version can actually be more filling and more nutritious.

Downsize your next meal to see how it works. If you downsize in a reasonable way in places that don't matter to you, you'll cut calories without feeling any loss at all.

Downsizing can also help you to get even more pleasure when you indulge yourself. I will never tell you to give up the things you love. I've read so many diet books that tell you, for example, to switch to skim milk in your coffee. What if you like cream in your coffee and you are going to be miserable with that watered-down beige coffee? I used to be that kind of person. I would lose my mind if I didn't have access to skim milk, as if cream were going to kill me. No skim milk, no coffee. It was idiotic.

Instead, downsizing lets you have the cream. Just have a little splash of cream in your coffee. It's no big deal as long as you aren't filling half your cup with half-and-half. I've seen obsessed women nearly have a nervous breakdown if they had accidentally tried a sip of sugared soda, and women who refuse to eat anything but fat-free, chemical-loaded peanut butter, fat-free salad dressings and mayo, and fat-free cookies instead of a downsized portion of the real thing. Do you see the absurdity? Do you see why downsizing makes so much sense? This rule will teach you how to eat whatever you want while never eating too much. And you'll never have to eat another bite of horrible, fake "diet food" again. What a relief!

HEAVY HABIT

Let's talk about peer pressure. I know I can tell you to eat less, but if you are with a group of your friends, and they are all eating huge portions, it can be really tough to break the mold and eat less. I recently read about a study that said women tend to weigh about the same as their friends, suggesting that groups of women develop similar eating habits. It's peer pressure, plain and simple.

But that doesn't mean you have to stop hanging out with your friends. Instead, just set a better example by not making food such a big deal (even if it is a big deal for your friends). You can still be fun, interesting, and the life of the party without gorging on pizza and beer, and if you focus on your friends and having a good time, you'll focus less on the food. If your friends are all eating a lot, fine. Let them. Have a slice and eat it very slowly so you aren't done before everyone else and staring at the remaining pizza. Have a beer, and sip it very slowly. Then stop. You might inspire your friends to notice and cut back, too. And if they tease you about your more moderate new habits? Just wait until they see you in your bikini or your new, downsized jeans.

No need to make a big deal about it. "I'm just not that hungry right now," is a perfectly nice answer. If you've had a healthy snack before you went out, you really won't be very hungry.

Your Downsizing Toolbox

I am not going to tell you to break out your measuring cups and spoons. You don't need these things to be naturally thin. In fact, most naturally thin people never measure anything unless they are cooking. Why should they measure? It's obsessive and it promotes the attitude that there is something wrong with you, as if, without special equipment, you are incapable of eating like a normal person. It's ridiculous, so stop it right now.

But just as I gave you a general idea about appropriate portions for common foods, I will tell you that having plates, bowls, and glasses in smaller sizes, plus a few key tools, will definitely help make downsizing easier. In this section, I'll show you exactly what I mean so you have a good idea of what is an appropriately sized dish to hold your popcorn, salad, or oatmeal. Don't sweat the cost if you don't have all of these items. You can buy most of the items in this chapter at Ikea or similar stores, such as 99¢ stores, for cheap.

Plates: When it comes to plates, size matters. If you put a little food on a big plate, you're going to feel cheated, even if you have plenty of food in front of you. But if you put your food on a plate that matches the amount of food, you'll feel you are getting the right amount. We eat with our eyes first, and first impressions make a difference in our eventual satisfaction. I always use a salad plate instead of a full-sized dinner plate for my meals and snacks at home. A dinner plate looks huge to me now, and an inappropriate size for the amount of food I usually choose to eat. So keep the salad plates at the front of your cabinet, and grab those first. Start serving dinner on them and everybody in your family will probably eat less without even noticing.

Bowls: Whenever I eat cereal, popcorn, or raw fruit, I use a small bowl. A Japanese rice bowl or a small cereal bowl is a great size for foods that aren't extremely calorie-dense. For foods like peanuts, chips, or ice cream, I use a ramekin (see below), but when it's appropriate to have a little more than that, a rice bowl makes more sense. A bowl of this size should comfortably hold about 1 cup of food. Never eat anything out of the bag—always use a bowl!

Ramekins: I consider these small—approximately ½ cup—ramekins or custard cups indispensable for downsizing. These little bowls are perfect for decadent treats like ice cream or chips. You fill them up but you still don't get too much food; you get just enough to satisfy you. I use these every day. If you don't have them, I suggest buying a set. They aren't very expensive, and you'll get more than your money's worth.

Small Casserole: If you frequently cook for just one or two people, it's a great idea to have a small casserole dish or an oval French baker. Many recipes make a huge amount. Why cook something that serves six to eight when you are cooking for only one to two? Cut the recipe in half, or make only a fourth of it, and use smaller baking pans. These pans are also great for heating up leftovers the next day, if you don't want to use the microwave. If you plan to buy one, try to find one with a lid, to make it even more versatile.

Muffin Tin: Instead of baking big cakes and loaves, bake cupcakes and muffins—automatic portion control. Mini muffin tins are great, too. (Avoid the tins that make the giant muffins.)

Juice and Dessert Wineglasses: Save the big tumblers and pint glasses for water. For juice, milk, and sugary drinks—and even beer—have just a little in a small juice glass. If you can pour just a little wine into a big wineglass, fine. You have more room for swirling and sniffing. But if you tend to fill those giant wineglasses, use the smaller glasses designed for dessert wines. You'll automatically drink less, but you'll still feel as if you had a glass of wine (because you did!).

Chopsticks: Although you can certainly use regular utensils, chopsticks are fun and can help slow you down, so you might want to try them instead once in a while. Plus, everybody wants to be adept at using chopsticks, right? Consider it good practice.

Microplane: A microplane is a tool for grating that results in very finely grated food. It's great for hard cheese (like Parmesan), chocolate, citrus peel, or spices (like nutmeg and cinnamon). Use it with spices for a very fresh flavor in baking. Use it with citrus to add fresh zest to recipes or drinks. Especially use it to add cheese or chocolate to foods without having to use very much. Unlike box graters, microplanes add just a dusting of flavor, so you'll get the impression of cheese or chocolate without piling on the calories and fat.

Immersion Blender: Pureed food is comforting and *filling*. It always makes me feel nurtured. But sometimes, a regular blender is just too unwieldy, especially for hot foods. Enter the immersion blender, a handy tool for pureeing right in the pan, bowl, or glass. Use it to make soup, sauces, fruit purees, and smoothies.

Freezer: Everybody has a freezer, but are you using yours to the best of your ability? I use a freezer in two important ways. First, I make homemade frozen dinners. If you have a big meal—let's use Thanksgiving as an example—you almost always have leftovers. Why not portion out individual small amounts of turkey, potatoes, vegetables, and pie? Warm these up when you are in a hurry, and you'll have something delicious and homemade instead of something processed and full of preservatives. I also freeze individual portions of homemade chili, soup, casseroles, and desserts. And speaking of desserts, this is the other way I use my freezer. It takes longer to eat frozen food, so freeze grapes, banana slices, mini Snickers bars, bite-sized brownie pieces, or small cookies. You'll have an easier time taking out a small portion and you'll be able to savor it more slowly.

Ice Cream Scoop: These scoops are great for portioning out more foods than just ice cream. You can also use them in baking to measure out batter for muffins, cupcakes, cookies, or crabcake batter. You can also portion out turkey burger meat or servings of mashed potatoes, rice, tuna, or chicken salad with this versatile tool.

Mini Chopper: This is perfect for chopping herbs, spices, and other flavorings like garlic and chocolate. These choppers aren't big or hard to break down or clean, so you can pull them out and use them whenever. They will encourage you to flavor your food more creatively.

Recyclable Plastic Containers: I have already mentioned food delivery services, but I can't help mentioning them again. If you have recyclable plastic containers handy, then every time you cook something or bring home leftovers, you can portion them out into downsized meals that you can put in your freezer and reheat at a moment's notice. I buy these in bulk at wholesale stores, including regular sizes for meals and small sizes for salad dressing. Why spend all that money on portion-controlled packaged food when you can have good homemade or restaurant food already portion-controlled in your freezer? These containers are invaluable for making that happen.

You can also use these containers for freezing individual portions of soup, or even for making salads and keeping them in the refrigerator. For example, buy a big bag of prewashed arugula, a few tomatoes, and just bang it out: make individual salads for the week, topping each one with a little leftover meat, a few nuts, or some cheese. This can save you a ton of money, and reduce waste. And when you bring a neat little plastic container to work, it looks chic, not sloppy. Your food will be all nicely arranged and fresh. (Bring the dressing in a separate small container so your salad doesn't get soggy. Drizzle it on just before eating.)

What's a Portion?

I don't like to tell people how much to eat. I'm never going to say to you, "Eat half a cup of broccoli and three ounces of chicken." What if you don't like broccoli? Or what if you want more broccoli? How much you eat depends on many things, not the least of which is how hungry you are at the moment. I think it's absurd to tell people how much to eat.

However, I also know what it's like to lose all sense of what a real portion is. To help *you* figure out for yourself how much you should eat, so you have a guide by which to measure whether you'd like a little less or a little more of something, here are some *approximate* reasonable sizes for some common food groups. Consider this a general guide. On some days, you will probably want a little more than this. On other days, half a portion might be more than enough. It all depends on what your food voice tells you.

Vegetables, Cooked: One portion of sautéed, steamed, boiled, or stir-fried vegetables would fill a small cereal bowl or salad plate. This is approximately ½ a cup to 1 cup. But to be perfectly honest, I've never measured my vegetables. They are *vegetables*! A big heap of them is a great investment.

Salad: One portion of raw leafy greens or lettuce with raw vegetables should fill a soup bowl or salad bowl, or be heaped on a salad plate. In general, a portion of raw vegetables is about two to three times bigger than a similar portion of cooked vegetables. If you must measure, a portion of salad is about 1 to 2 cups. Dress lightly with dressing, don't drown your lettuce, but don't worry about measuring out your dressing—that's obsessive.

Raw Fruit: One medium-sized piece of fruit, like an apple, pear, or peach, is a portion. Two plums or two apricots are a portion. For berries or chopped fruit like melons, aim to fill a small cereal bowl (about the size of half of a grapefruit) or Japanese rice bowl, or about 1 cup. But please don't stress about measuring or weighing your fruit. I hate it when diet books say, "Eat a *small* apple." Maybe I want a *big* apple. It's an *apple*. It's not going to make you fat.

Meat, Poultry, and Fish: A portion is a piece of meat, poultry, or fish about the size of a small kitchen sponge. If it's really fatty, make it a little smaller, maybe the size of a cell phone. If it's really lean, you can make it a little bigger.

Pasta and Rice: A small Japanese rice bowl is the right size for a portion of pasta or rice. It doesn't sound like much, and sometimes you might want more, but remember that white pasta and white rice are likely to make you even hungrier, so they aren't very good investments. Fill the bowl level, don't heap it full.

Cereal: If it's full of bran and made with whole grains and little or no sugar, fill a Japanese rice bowl or small cereal bowl about two-thirds full. If the cereal is puffy and sugary—well, are you sure you really want it? If you do, fill the bowl only about half of the way. No refilling it just to finish up the milk!

Bread: One medium-sized slice, half a scooped bagel, half a scooped English muffin, or one small dinner roll is a portion. By "scooped," I mean that I pull out some of the bread and throw it away. I'll talk more about this in Chapter 15. By the way, if the bread, bagel, or roll is gigantic, you know perfectly well that's two or three portions. Can you split it with somebody?

Muffins, Cookies, and Pastries: The same thing applies to muffins, cookies, and pastries as to bread. If it's medium-sized, it's a portion. If it's gigantic, it should not be for one person. Split it or save half for later.

Cheese: A piece of cheese the size of a business card. I'm a fan of soy cheese slices on sandwiches. Obviously, one slice is a portion.

Ice Cream: One scoop in a ramekin or custard cup is a portion. Nobody needs more than one small scoop of ice cream in a day.

Popcorn: Popcorn in a larger cereal or rice bowl is a portion. If you put butter on it, that also counts as a portion of fat. Don't use very much. The popcorn shouldn't be swimming.

Chips, Crackers, and Pretzels: A small ramekin of chips or crackers should be plenty, even if the bag says a portion is twelve or twenty or whatever. Just get a taste of the crunchiness and stop. But you don't have to count.

Nuts: A small handful, unless you have large hands, and I don't mean a handful so big that nuts are falling out between your fingers. I'm talking about approximately ¼ cup. But a small serving of nuts makes an excellent snack that will stick with you. If you use a ramekin, fill it only about halfway.

Nut Butter, Hummus, Guacamole: A thin spread. You don't need to measure. Just don't glop it on. Use your common sense and don't lie to yourself.

Juice: If you like juice (I do), don't be deterred by people who say you should never drink it. Obviously, whole fruit is better because of the fiber, which is filling and good for you, but if you really want juice, have some in a small juice glass or small wineglass. I like to mix mine with sparkling water. You don't need to fill up a big water glass—that's too much sugar. It's natural sugar, but it's still sugar. The bottom line is, there is no forbidden food—but I'll hold back somewhere else if I want juice. Make your choice.

HEAVY HABIT

I've noticed a trend to join food delivery services. In fact, a lot of big companies are making a lot of money by doing your downsizing for you—for a hefty fee! It's all about portion control. You can't do that yourself? I've tried these food delivery services, and I know they make you feel you are getting away with something because they often send decadent foods that you wouldn't normally let yourself eat, like pancakes and sausage. The trick is that these foods come in small portions, so anyone could eat them and lose weight. The delivery service makes you think there is some secret involved, but if you eat one small pancake, a little syrup, and one sausage, then you aren't going to get fat. Why not just make your own meals by putting leftovers together in plastic storage containers, labeling them with what's inside, and freezing them? You'll save money, the food will be less processed, and you'll get naturally thin because you controlled your portions on your own. Like a grown-up. For free.

Wine or Beer: A small glass of wine, or half a bottle of beer, is a portion. Don't kid yourself.

Liquor: One shot is a portion. Stick with clear liquor and use mixers that aren't loaded with sugar, like seltzer or freshly squeezed fruit juice.

It's Not about Measuring

Finally, I want to emphasize again that I do not want you to measure your food. One of the most important points I want you to take away from this book is that you can eat like a normal, naturally thin person. You aren't on a diet. You aren't deprived or required to eat differently. You aren't eating obsessively or with anxiety and worry. Instead, choose to downsize, but do it in a sensible, non-obsessive way.

So use small plates, bowls, and glasses. Don't feel compelled to finish every bite. Pay attention to how you feel, and listen to your food voice to know what you really want and when you've had enough.

If you sit there with your measuring spoons, angry at the world that you have to do this because you need to lose weight, you won't be happy and you probably won't lose weight, or if you do, it won't stay lost. Eventually, you will rebel and eat too much, out of deprivation and desperation.

But when you learn how to downsize naturally and normally with intention, purpose, and forethought, you *will* become naturally thin, and you won't be missing a thing.

Rule 5 Recipes

These easy, delicious recipes are custom-made to come in small portions.

Classic Crab Cakes

I love crab cakes and I often order appetizer portions of crab cakes in restaurants, but you can make them at home, too. When you use a nonstick pan and cooking spray, you significantly reduce the fat content, compared with crab cakes that are fried in oil.

Makes 12 large crabcakes, or 24 small

2 tablespoons olive oil

¾ cup small-diced red onion

1½ cups small-diced celery

1½ cups of each: small-diced red and yellow bell pepper

1½ teaspoons Old Bay seasoning

½ teaspoon salt

½ teaspoon ground black pepper

½ cup whole wheat bread crumbs (preferably panko)

¼ cup lowfat mayonnaise or soy mayonnaise (I like Nayonnaise brand)

2 teaspoons Dijon mustard

1 teaspoon Worcestershire sauce

½ pound (8 ounces) jumbo lump crabmeat, drained

Cooking spray

2 tablespoons store-bought pesto + 2 tablespoons lowfat mayonnaise (or soy mayonnaise) mixed together and seasoned with salt and pepper to taste

2 tablespoons fresh minced parsley

1. Heat the oil in a pan and sauté the onion, celery, and bell peppers until soft. Season with Old Bay, salt, and pepper. Set aside to cool.

2. In a large bowl, combine the bread crumbs, mayonnaise, mustard, and Worcestershire sauce. Stir in the crabmeat to combine but don't overmix. The crabmeat should remain in large pieces. Combine ingredients from steps 1 and 2.

3. Spray a nonstick pan with cooking spray and turn heat to medium. Scoop evenly-sized cakes into the pan using an ice cream scoop and sauté over medium heat until crispy on both sides. Top each crab cake with tiny dab of pesto/mayonnaise mixture. Sprinkle with parsley and serve immediately.

Coconut Cupcakes

I make these vegan cupcakes for my company, BethennyBakes, and they are to die for . . . if you are one of those people who loves coconut. If you don't like coconut, just leave it out.

Makes 8 cupcakes

¾ cup raw sugar

1¼ cups oat flour

⅓ cup vegan shortening (mixed into the flour, not melted)

1½ teaspoons baking powder

½ teaspoon salt

½ cup soymilk

¾ teaspoon vanilla extract

¾ teaspoon coconut extract

1. Preheat the oven to 350°F. Line cupcake pans with liners.
2. Combine all the dry ingredients in one bowl and all the wet ingredients in another. Mix them each, then mix them together.
3. Using an ice cream scoop (perfect for portion control), transfer the batter into the liners. Bake for 20 minutes, rotating the pan after 10 minutes, or until tops of cupcakes are firm. Let cool.

Coconut Icing

½ cup vegan shortening

½ cup vegan margarine

3½ cups powdered sugar

1½ teaspoons vanilla extract

½ teaspoon coconut extract

Shaved coconut for garnish (about 1 cup)

Mix all ingredients together, then spread on the cupcakes. Garnish with shaved coconut.

Chapter 6

CANCEL YOUR MEMBERSHIP IN THE CLEAN PLATE CLUB

Put the fork down, already. They have dishwashers for that.

This rule is about your plate, and what you choose to leave on it. I know some of you are used to finishing everything on your plate. Waste not, want not, right? Well, those days are over. But so are the days of desperation, feeling sick and a little disappointed in yourself when you see your shiny clean plate and the plates of others who don't even seem to notice that they have left half a sandwich or most of their fries. That can be you. You just have to decide that it is you.

This brings us to rule 6:

❦ Cancel your membership in the Clean Plate Club. ❦

Leaving some food on your plate sounds easy, but it is actually difficult if you aren't in the habit. You might not even realize you have finished it all until it's gone (probably partly because you didn't *pay attention* when you were eating). But this rule is going to help you change all that, by employing some very specific strategies that will help you feel less obsessed about the food on your plate, less attached to it, and more able to let it go somewhere else.

This simple rule has impressive power, even though I'm telling you to go against your mother's advice. But our world is different from the one your mother or grandmother lived in, when food was scarce and every bite was precious. Today, food is—for better or for worse—plentiful, not to mention a lot less natural than it used to be.

This rule isn't about wasting food. On the contrary, this chapter will help you get *more* for your money by making one meal into several meals, by increasing the fun factor in meals, and by putting less food into your body. I am giving you some strategies to keep from eating more food than you really want to eat. I want you to be able to look at a big plate of food in a restaurant and know how to handle it without panicking over finishing it all or how much you should have or whether it's OK to eat at all. I want you to calm down, listen to your food voice, eat a little bit of it, and then *share it, save it, or leave it.*

Rule 6 is particularly valuable in restaurants. I eat out often (and I know that a lot of you do, too), and I invoke this rule all the time. If I'm at home having a piece of toast, I don't worry about leaving any of it. I'll eat it all. It's just a piece of toast. But in a restaurant with all that rich food and those huge portions, and everybody at the table ordering something different, this rule comes in handy. You need a strategy and a plan, and this rule is it.

You can practice this rule in three main ways, so I'll talk about them separately before I bring them together. Let's start with sharing.

HEAVY HABIT

Are you a person who stops everything the second the food arrives and focuses entirely on eating? Well, stop it. It's just rude, for one thing. And think about it: is food really that important? You can relish and enjoy every bite of your food without acting as if you are having the last meal of your life. If you focus on the company, the conversation, the environment, the atmosphere, and having a calm and relaxing time, you will have a much better experience, and enjoy your food even more. Balance your dining experience. It's not all about the food.

Share Your Food

You've got a lot of food in front of you, and a lot of people at your table. How do you make the evening more fun, bring everyone together, and limit your portion of food at the same time?

Share your food. Sharing food helps you eat less while allowing you to taste more. Everybody at the table gets to sample more of what a restaurant has to offer. Whenever I order something in a restaurant—salad, appetizer, soup, entrée, even a drink—I always offer a taste of it to whomever I'm with. Sometimes nobody takes me up on the offer to taste what I've ordered, but more often than not, people are curious about food and happy to have just a taste of what someone else chose. It's fun to taste a lot of different food. By giving others that opportunity, you become a more interesting dinner companion, and more fun. Sharing fosters a sense of togetherness at the table and helps everybody feel more in tune with everybody else.

You don't have to be in a big group of people to share. When I go out on a date, for example, we often share, and that makes dinner more of an experience. It usually works like this. Together, we choose a salad, an entrée, an appetizer, and a couple of side dishes. If my date likes steak, I usually have just a couple of bites of the steak, and he eats the rest. I love appetizers like crab cakes and calamari, so I usually get one of those. He has a few bites of the appetizer, so I never end up eating the whole thing. We usually split the salad, each eating about half. The side dishes—for example, sautéed mushrooms, broccoli rabe, or a baked potato—we also split, so we both get to fill up on fiber-rich vegetables. If we decide to get dessert, I take a couple of bites. We don't always get dessert, but it's certainly not forbidden. This is just an example of how a date sometimes goes, but do you see how sharing can make a meal more of an event? It can also make a date more intimate or friendly.

The sharing contributes to the feeling of being on a date and nobody feels deprived, but when you add it up, each person actually eats a lot less than they might have. This is the SkinnyGirl mentality.

NATURALLY THIN THOUGHT

Some restaurants charge you extra for sharing because they would rather have you order two entrées. Of course they would. They make more money that way, and the server gets a bigger tip. But why should you pay for food you don't want? To get around this, don't ask for an additional plate for sharing. Instead, one of you can order an entrée and a salad, and the other can order an appetizer as an entrée, and soup or a side dish. Then you can both share from each other's plates without raising any eyebrows. Besides, it's more romantic that way.

Dieting Is Anti-Sharing

Dieting is the antithesis of sharing. When you are on a diet, it's hard to share. Your portions are so small and the meager bits of food you get—food you may not really even like—seem like a lifeboat you must cling to in order to survive. You guard it almost jealously!

If you get only half a cup of brown rice and three ounces of skinless chicken, you certainly aren't going to want to share it. You need every bite! (Never mind that you're going to go crazy and eat a pint of ice cream later in the night because you are starving and feel deprived.)

But that's not you (anymore), because you are so over dieting. When you can order anything you want, and you give yourself permission to get maximum pleasure out of your food, of course you want to share that abundance. You've got salad and soup, crab cakes, and a SkinnyGirl Margarita in front of you. Share the wealth!

Sharing is also a great way to help you learn when you are full. If you aren't yet in the habit of recognizing when you've had enough food, or of specifically identifying your *point of diminishing returns* (the point when you've extracted the maximum enjoyment from your food, so you might as well stop eating), sharing helps you get some of that food off your plate. Every bite you share is a bite you don't eat, so sharing helps your body get used to the feeling of eating less, while getting to try more foods. That's when you start to recognize that less really is more. See, your mother *was* right when she told you that sharing is a virtue.

Save It

I don't like to waste good food, and in this time of global environmental consciousness, rising food prices, and fuel shortages, I think it's irresponsible. I want to help conserve our planet's resources, and you probably do, too. So what do you do if nobody else wants the food on your plate but you know you've already had enough?

Save it.

I often take food home in a doggie bag, but not for my dog, Cookie. I love having a beautiful, healthy, delicious lunch or dinner to look forward to the next day. It is economical, it is figure-friendly, and it gives you one less meal to plan the day after. A few small pieces of leftover steak sliced thinly over greens, sprinkled with cheese and a light vinaigrette, are a beautiful lunch. Otherwise, the leftovers would be in the garbage.

Never feel embarrassed to take food home!

Remember: the doggie isn't the one who takes the bag home, but the one who finishes everything on the plate. Do you really want to eat like a dog? No—I don't either.

Another reason to save leftovers is to combine two concepts: *save it* and *share it*. If you have kids, they might love to get a taste of the evening out that they missed, and they'll get a taste by feasting on your leftovers. Your boyfriend or husband might enjoy leftovers if he missed the girls'-night-out dinner.

And of course, your dog really might want some of those leftovers, too. Just a little, now. You don't want your dog getting too fat either.

What if you are one of those people who just can't leave half your food? Practice prevention by asking the server to pack up half the entree in a doggie back before you even see it. Instant portion control!

NATURALLY THIN THOUGHT

- Salads are a great way to use leftover steak, chicken, or fish. For example, slice leftover steak and arrange it over a bed of fresh arugula, lightly dressed with your favorite dressing, for a delicious sliced steak salad.
- Toss broccoli rabe, spinach, or any other vegetable from the night before with crumbled turkey sausage, hot cooked whole-wheat pasta, and toasted pine nuts for an entirely new dish.
- Even a tiny bit of leftover sautéed mushrooms or onions can become a great frittata the next day.

The more creative you are, the more inspired you will be to save part of your meal for the next day. You're getting two great meals for the price of one.

Leave It

What can you do if you order something, you share some, you eat some, and suddenly you realize that the food *really isn't all that good*? Or maybe the food is fine but you really can't take it home with you because you won't be in a situation where you can carry it or store it safely. You've eaten enough and you have a quarter of your food left. What should you do?

Leave it.

Leaving food on your plate is *not* wasting food.

Forget all those stories about starving children. You can't send your food to them. Leaving some food on your plate is an easy, effective way to eat less. If you eat what you want to eat but leave some, you won't feel deprived, and you'll also be exercising your own will: you decide you've had enough, so you stop before it's all gone. The food isn't controlling you. You are controlling how much you eat. That's a great feeling, and it's what naturally thin people do.

Eating food you don't want and making yourself fatter is the real waste—a waste of your health and your life energy, not to mention a waste of money.

Here's my general policy: If I eat a small portion of something really decadent, like ice cream, cake, or chips, I always try to leave at least two bites. If I order something large, like an entrée or a big muffin at a bakery, I try to leave half (often sharing it with someone or saving half for later). If I order something that I consider a good investment but the portion is quite big, I try to leave a quarter of it on my plate.

But don't worry about the numbers. You can start this process by simply leaving one or two bites of something you would normally finish. When you are comfortable with that, gradually increase the amount you leave. If you have always been a tried-and-true member of the Clean Plate Club, canceling your membership will be a big step and leaving just one bite will be great progress.

How much I leave varies, and these aren't hard-and-fast rules, but

I always try to leave something, and the way I determine how much is often a matter of when my food voice tells me I've had enough. 🍷 *Pay attention* 🍷 and you'll soon learn to recognize when you really would rather leave more, or a little less. Save it if it's enough to save. If it's not, leave it. Don't eat if you don't really want it, or if you've already passed the *point of diminishing returns*.

Think of it this way: eating a whole huge plate of food because you "hate to waste" is a waste of *you*. Drop the baggage and let it go. Leaving food that you can't share and don't want to save because it really wasn't that good is *not* a waste. It's the only rational choice.

When You Just Can't Do It

I know. Sometimes it's really hard to leave food on your plate. You're extra hungry, or the food tastes so good that you find it extremely difficult to stop eating. Some days, you'll find it easy to leave two bites or a quarter or half of your food. You'll have no problem sharing, saving, or leaving it.

If you are one of those people who simply can't leave food on your plate (but keep in mind that you may not always be one of those people—you may change) or you just happen to be particularly hungry (we all have those days), you need to be the perfect eater. This means that you order very carefully. Maybe you'll have a glass of wine, a low-calorie salad, and a simple grilled entrée with no bread, dessert, or extras. If that's how you like to eat, great. If you need to finish everything, do it. Personally, as a rule, I prefer to taste more things and not finish them, rather than be so Spartan in my choices. But it all depends on you. Only you know what you need and want to do. You might not like eating the way I do, and that's fine. However you like to eat, you can be naturally thin.

And what if you don't order perfectly, and you finish everything anyway? Well, that's life. We all overdo it on occasion.

Don't beat yourself up. You're only human. It will do more harm than good to hate yourself and feel guilty. Then you're more likely to do it again. Every now and then, I make the same mistake, eating more than I wanted to eat. But the point is not to let this get you off track. Shrug it off and go light on the next meal with healthy, energizing choices like vegetables and lean protein. You'll be fine. Next time, you'll share it, save it, or leave it. The trick is not to make this a habit or get angry at yourself. These little slipups should be the exception, not the norm. You'll know you ate too much when you feel too full, bloated, and low on energy. The beauty of sharing, saving, or leaving food is that you can eat what you want but still feel light and energetic, not tired and heavy.

When you overindulge, notice how you feel the next day, and that will also tell you something. If you feel bloated and sluggish, if your ankles are swollen, and if you can't get your rings on, you'll know you overdid it. If you feel light, energetic, and clean, you'll know you got it right. Remember that wonderful feeling. It's worth making smart choices to have this feeling more often, and that means you need to *cancel your membership in the Clean Plate Club,* and cancel it now.

Rule 6 Recipes

Beautiful, rich food is easy to overeat, but when you make it in small portions, you'll have an easier time putting on the brakes. These rich recipes are portioned, but that doesn't mean you can't still share, save some, or leave some.

Classic Zucchini Soufflé

These gorgeous little soufflés are great to serve guests, but you can also make them at home for your family, just because you want to serve them something special. Baking them in individual ramekins helps you control portions—these are rich! They are small, but that doesn't mean you can't still leave two bites. Serve this with a big beautiful salad, so you fill up on raw vegetables.

Serves 6

4 cups shredded zucchini

1¼ teaspoons salt

1 tablespoon melted butter

4 eggs

1 teaspoon fresh thyme, chopped

⅛ teaspoon ground black pepper

Pinch of red pepper flakes

1 cup shredded Monterey Jack cheese

1 tablespoon grated Parmesan

¼ cup all-purpose biscuit baking mix

1. Toss the zucchini and salt together and place into a colander set in the sink. Allow to drain for 1 hour, then squeeze the liquid out of the zucchini, and set aside.

2. Preheat oven to 350°F. Brush a 6-cup muffin tin, or 6 individual ramekins, with the butter

3. Whisk the eggs in a mixing bowl with the thyme, pepper, and red pepper flakes. Stir in the zucchini, Monterey Jack cheese, Parmesan, and baking mix, until combined. Pour into the prepared muffin tin or ramekins.

4. Bake, uncovered, until set and golden brown on top, about 20 minutes. The soufflé is done when a knife inserted into the center comes out clean.

Joyful Heart Muffins

I created these low-fat, wheat-free, dairy-free fudgy chocolate chip muffins for Mariska Hargitay, who cofounded the Joyful Heart Foundation. Mariska is an actress who has won the Golden Globe and Emmy awards, and a very dear friend of mine.

Serves 8

Nonstick cooking spray

1 cup unsweetened applesauce

½ cup raw sugar

1 teaspoon vanilla

1 teaspoon almond extract

1 teaspoon canola oil

¾ cup oat flour (to make oat flour, pulverize dry rolled oats to a powder in a blender)

⅓ cup unsweetened cocoa powder

2 teaspoons baking powder

½ teaspoon baking soda

½ teaspoon salt

Dash of cinnamon

½ cup semisweet vegan chocolate chips

1. Preheat the oven to 375°F. Spray a regular-sized muffin tin with cooking spray. If you have only a muffin tin that holds 12 muffins, use just 8 of the cups.

2. In a small bowl, combine the applesauce, sugar, vanilla, almond extract, and canola oil. Stir and set aside to allow the sugar crystals to dissolve.

3. In a large bowl, sift together the oat flour, cocoa powder, baking powder, baking soda, salt, and cinnamon. If you don't want to take the time to sift, mix them well with a wire whisk to aerate the dry ingredients.

4. Add the applesauce mixture to the flour mixture and stir until combined. Fold in chocolate chips.

5. Using a 3-ounce ice cream scoop or a large spoon, divide the batter between 8 muffin cups. Bake for 20 minutes, or until the tops are firm to the touch.

6. Cool completely on a wire rack, then pop the muffins out with a spoon.

Chapter 7

CHECK YOURSELF BEFORE
YOU WRECK YOURSELF

What I'm about to tell you in this chapter changed my life. Every rule in this book is important, but rule 7 is important in a deeply personal way. If binge-eating is a problem for you, this chapter might just change your life, too. It is about binging, which I call *wrecking yourself*. It's something I used to do, but it's something I *never* do anymore. *And I mean never.*

I'm not going to talk about any celebrities in this chapter, because who is and isn't binging is a personal matter—and I feel really comfortable talking only about myself with regard to this sensitive subject. It's what rule 7 is all about:

Check yourself before you wreck yourself.

In other words, stop yourself before you binge. But of course, this is easier said than done, so let's talk about binging.

Binging versus Overeating

Binging is different from overeating. Everybody overeats now and then. It's part of living. On special occasions, on particularly hungry days, or when you have PMS, you know what I mean. It's a holiday a party, or you didn't get a chance to have lunch. For whatever reason, sometimes you eat more than you do at other times. Sometimes you even eat more than you really want to eat.

But binging is more extreme. When you binge, you lose control of your behavior. The food takes over and you eat *much* more than you know you should eat, but you feel that you can't help it. Sometimes you feel that you are in so deep there is no turning back. The food takes precedence over anything else, until you are done. Then you feel overwhelmed by guilt, helplessness, anger, self-loathing. So you do it again, caught in a vicious cycle of binging, guilt, regret, and more binging. If you've ever done this, you know what I'm talking about.

I've binged in the past. I never purged, and I was not bulimic—and if you have this problem, please seek professional help, because it can be very difficult to overcome on your own. In my case, binging was more of a bad habit.

As a single girl living in Manhattan, I found it particularly difficult to avoid binging. I can't tell you how many times I would come home late at night after going out with my friends. Many times, I skipped dinner because I was having a few drinks or moving from place to place and never had time to eat, or I couldn't afford to eat out. I wouldn't think about the consequences until I got home, starving.

That's when I would pass a bodega or a deli and I wouldn't know what I wanted, so I'd get everything. I remember once buying a bag of Ruffles, a pint of ice cream, and one of those giant muffins the size of a small house. I went inside and I ate it all. I was like an automatic tennis ball machine.

The next day, I had a food hangover. I had a headache, my eyes were swollen, and the rest of me was swollen, too. Do you know this feeling? You feel like an animal. You vow never to eat again. It's happened to me what feels like a million times. I exaggerate, of course, but you know what I mean. You have a slice of pizza, and suddenly it's not enough, and you have two more slices, and then you need ice cream, cookies, and anything else you can find. Food is all you can focus on. Sometimes a binge starts in the morning, and you obsess all day. And then you want a do over. You wish you could take the whole day back.

But you can't. In life, you don't get a do-over. You just do. So this is your chance to start doing it right.

Why Binge?

I think binging happens for more than one reason. First, I think that for some people, binging may stem from a feeling of deprivation. You diet, you deprive yourself of foods you really want, you subsist on inferior substitutes like frozen diet meals and fat-free junk food, and finally you just can't take it anymore. Your body is crying out for something more, something real, and you don't know what it is, so you eat everything in a desperate attempt to find what's missing.

I'm not a nutritionist, but I believe this feeling of deprivation may have a physical component. If you eat a lot of fake food and not much real, whole food, you are probably missing out on hundreds of major and minor nutrients (antioxidants, fatty acids, phytochemicals, etc.), perhaps even some that nutrition science hasn't yet discovered. Whole foods, I strongly suspect, contain more than just the sum of their parts broken down, chemically synthesized, and packaged for microwaving. Our bodies aren't designed to eat fake food. We're designed to eat real food (rule 9 is about this). Go too long eating too little real food and too few calories, and pile on feelings of deprivation as you continually deny your impulses and shut down your pleasure centers, and bam—you've set yourself up for a binge.

This is why I believe in eating what you want, and choosing real food, so your body knows what it is getting and feels satiated.

But I think the key to binging goes beyond the physical. The mind and body are linked, and emotional denial can lead to a physical backlash. I believe the emotional component of binging is deeply rooted in a dysfunctional relationship with food. Nobody is ever genuinely hungry enough to eat as much food as people eat during a binge. But it's as though a switch goes off, and you eat like a motor. There is obviously something else going on when your brain shuts down like this. If you have a love-hate relationship with food, based on fear and obsession, binging can become the unhappy consummation of that dysfunctional relationship.

Before I get into my own experience, I need to make a disclaimer. If you have an eating disorder, you might not be able to fix it yourself. It doesn't mean there is anything wrong with you. You aren't weak or incapable. Eating disorders can be caused by serious medical or psychological imbalances (or both), and there are qualified medical professionals who can help you. I'm not a medical professional, so if you feel that you need help with an eating disorder, especially if you purge or starve yourself or really feel you can't do anything about your eating disorder on your own, please get help. Talk to your doctor about it, and don't delay. Don't waste any more time fearing, hating, and obsessing about food.

But in some cases, you may be able to get a handle on this by yourself, the way I did. If this is you, or you think it might be, I'll tell you how I did it. I want to set you on the path to discovering how you can improve *your* relationship with food, so you never have to waste another day immersed in negative food thoughts. I want you to be able to enjoy food and not be chained to it like a prisoner. It is possible to get there. I know, because I did it.

For me, binging was intimately tied up with a fear of food.

I used to fear french fries. I feared cookies. I feared steak, candy bars, and ice cream. I even feared avocado. I'd ask for my sushi rolls without avocado so I wouldn't have that fat. I was afraid of eating avocado. Somehow, I convinced myself that eating even one bite of avocado would make me fat, so I avoided it like the plague. Today, this seems ridiculous to me, but I remember feeling this way and it was very real to me at the time.

At the same time, I was also obsessed with food. I used it for comfort and to dull strong emotions. It took me a long time to realize that food was not my friend or my enemy.

Now, I eat avocado. I eat steak, ice cream, and even french fries. I'm not afraid of food anymore, and my relationship with foods—all foods—has normalized. Naturally thin people aren't afraid of french fries. So why was I? Why are you? When I figured this out, I stopped binging.

Stop Binging

It's easy for me to say, "Stop binging," but I realize it's a lot harder to actually stop if you are in the habit of emotional eating. You have to decide to stop doing this. You have to *break the habit*. Let's look at some of the good reasons why you should never binge again.

First, let's be pragmatic. Consider the math. If you added up the calories in a day of eating normal portions of what you want, versus a day of deprivation and a binge, you'd see that the binge day always comes out higher. Eating what you want most of the time and sometimes binging sounds better but also will put you over the top. If you are eating what you want, there is never a reason to binge, so just stop. Don't do it. It doesn't add up. It's right there in the numbers.

One binge may not make you fat, but habitual binging will. I like to say that no food is forbidden. But binging *should be* forbidden. I want you to take care of yourself, and binging is no way to do that.

Now, I'm a big fan of indulging myself, and I'm certainly not saying you shouldn't ever indulge yourself again. But indulging is completely different from binging. If you indulge yourself in the foods you love, you won't ever have to binge. You won't be desperate. You'll be well fed.

Listen to me. Food isn't a dark evil force out to get you and make you fat. It's not your best friend or your enemy. It's also not your girl-friend who will always be there for you when you are feeling stressed out, depressed, or emotional. It doesn't love you and it doesn't hate you. It's *food*. I know this sounds obvious, but sometimes, it helps to remind yourself, and that will help you ♡ *check yourself before you wreck yourself.* ♡

NATURALLY THIN THOUGHT

Some foods naturally flush water out of your system when you feel bloated from overeating. When you need to take it easy, focus on these de-bloating foods:

- Melons (especially cantaloupe)
- Asparagus
- Cucumbers
- Apple cider vinegar
- Celery

That's not to say there isn't an emotional component to food. Most people use food for comfort, and denying this truth can set you up for a binge. Instead, you can recognize that sometimes you are going to eat for emotional reasons, and then you can do it *consciously*, without binging. Emotional eating is not the same as binging, but it can lead to binging if you let the emotions take over. If you decide to eat for emotional reasons, do it with forethought. Decide what you will eat, portion it out, and stick with that. Then, enjoy it. Let it heal you, but don't forget that it really is only food. When you recognize that french fries aren't the enemy, that they are just food, you've taken the first step toward being able to eat a few and move on with your life. The old me would eat fries and feel so guilty that I'd eat them all, almost in a panic. Now, I never get to that point anymore. I always know I can stop, and I always know there will be plenty of other chances to eat french fries again. I quit my bad habit by recognizing that it's OK to eat, but it's not OK to hurt myself with food.

Binging is self-loathing, anxiety-producing, and bloating, with no upside. The notion that you can fix a binge the next day by fasting is misguided and ridiculous. Binges take days to correct, they are very hard on your body, and they stress you out mentally and emotionally. Instead, be present. Live in the moment. When you eat fattening food, fine. It happened. You're still a good person. Now, move on to the next moment and resume your healthy lifestyle, rather than dwelling on your lapse and falling into a pit of despair that will make you binge again.

Remember that life is a bunch of connected hours and days. Sometimes you will eat more; sometimes you will eat less. That's the way it is. But every time you choose to eat something, you have a new chance to make a good investment. Don't waste your hours and days on guilt and binging. Don't plan to "be good tomorrow." Be good to yourself *now*, and always. You don't need to live in a pit of despair, and you don't need to punish yourself. I'm serious about this. *Never binge again.*

NATURALLY THIN THOUGHT

I practice yoga, in which there is a principle called *ahimsa*, meaning non-violence. Beyond the obvious sense of not hurting others, this principle also applies to what you do to yourself. Binging hurts you, so practice *ahimsa* and be good to yourself by giving up binging for good.

Coming Out on the Other Side

It's a great feeling when you first learn how to stop binging, especially when you recognize that you are in a situation where you *might have binged, but didn't.* When you can taste something good and stop, or when you decide not to eat at a certain moment because you are particularly anxious, or when you learn to fill up on healthful food first and they calmly and happily enjoy something that once would have triggered a binge, you'll know you've made a huge step in the right direction.

Follow me here. I'm not afraid of avocados anymore. I don't mainline them, either. Avocados are no scarier to me than any other food. Now I see how people identify, weirdly, things they think they can and can't eat, like cream or salad dressing. I'm in control of avocados because I'm in control of myself, and because no food is off-limits. So I'm not afraid anymore. I take a few bites because I know I'll see this food again. I know that it's not forbidden, that I'm allowed to eat it.

Sure, some days I eat like a ravenous animal early in the day. By lunch, I've eaten enough calories to fill a whole day of sensible eating. I'm never thrilled about this, but I also see it as a challenge to let my body relax and recharge for the rest of the day without overburdening it anymore. I ate a lot because on that day, I felt I needed it. Most of the time, the next day is often completely different—I'll wake up and not be hungry at all until lunchtime.

During periods of stress, extensive travel, changes in the weather, changes at work, and other ups and downs, your eating habits *will* change. There is nothing wrong with that. You aren't the same every day—nobody is. Listen to your body. Listening is part of any healthy relationship. The best way to handle changes is to accept them, go with them, manage them to the best of your ability, and move on. If you have to obsess about something (I know I do), then obsess about more important things—cleaning your house, wearing a great outfit, surfing, accessorizing, long-distance running, finally writing the story of your life, or whatever it is.

If you make just one single change in your life based on reading this book, if you absorb only one thing, then make it this one: *never binge*. I know from personal experience that never binging again is not only *entirely possible*, but *absolutely life-changing*.

Moving Toward Peace

If you need to, it's time for you to make your own peace with food. The journey toward a healthy relationship with food can start today, but it won't end today. Be kind to yourself, and if you slip up and wreck yourself with a binge, forgive yourself so that you don't make it any worse. Step back and look at where you are going and what role you want food to play in your life, and then gently return to the path. If you've been unkind to yourself by binging, you need even more nurturing, not less. Treat yourself even *better* than usual, not worse. No punishment!

And if you slipped up and ate too much and now you feel horrible, try the following recipes, which can help you recover from a binge. They are cleansing, calming, and kind. I call them "recovery" recipes. (I'm working on a book all about cleansing, so keep an eye out for that.)

Rule 7 Recovery Recipes

If you overdid it and you feel bloated and horrible, don't focus on your guilt—focus on healing. Treat yourself gently and eat gentle, cleansing, easily digestible foods that will naturally flush excess water from your system and make you feel better. These are also good whenever you feel like eating more lightly, even if you haven't binged.

Pureed Zucchini Soup

The perfect, gentle, purifying, savory, delicious soup, this will make you feel better whenever you eat it.

Serves 6 to 8

1 medium red onion, evenly chopped
Nonstick cooking spray

6 cups chicken stock or broth

6 medium-sized zucchini, evenly chopped

Salt and pepper, to taste

12 oz. frozen butternut squash, defrosted

1 cup plain soymilk

Juice of ½ a lemon

1. Sauté the onions in a large pot using nonstick cooking spray, until slightly soft. Add the chicken stock or broth, zucchini, salt, and pepper. Cook until zucchini are soft.

2. Using a hand (immersion) blender, puree the onion-zucchini mixture until smooth. Add the defrosted butternut squash. Turn off the heat and add the soymilk and lemon juice. Season with more salt and pepper, to taste.

Cool Cucumber Salad

Cucumbers are a natural diuretic, and this fresh cold salad is perfect for hot, humid days when you feel not only bloated but sweaty and uncomfortable.

Serves 1 (but you can multiply it for more people)

1 medium cucumber

¼ cup apple cider vinegar

1 tablespoon chopped fresh dill, plus sprigs for garnish (or your favorite herb)

1 teaspoon honey

1 teaspoon lemon juice

Salt and pepper, to taste

1. Peel and thinly slice the cucumber. Put the slices in a bowl and set aside.

2. In a separate bowl, whisk together the vinegar, dill, honey, and lemon juice. Pour over the cucumbers and toss to coat. Season with a little salt and pepper.

3. Cover with a lid or plastic wrap and refrigerate for at least 30 minutes to chill and incorporate the flavors. Enjoy this salad cold. Garnish with a few extra sprigs of fresh dill.

Chapter 8

KNOW THYSELF

I can't overstate the importance of rule 8, because most diet plans overlook it. They tell you what to eat. They tell you how to exercise, and for how long. They tell you exactly what you need to do to lose weight.

Do they know you?

Of course they don't. Maybe that explains why diets so often fail. I don't care how famous the person is who is touting the latest diet. I don't care how many promises authors make on the covers of their books. You are you, and only *you* know what you like to eat, how you like to exercise, and what kind of life you prefer.

How can anybody else really know you better than you know yourself? If you want to be naturally thin, you have a responsibility to know yourself. If you don't feel that you know or understand yourself very well, it's time to get acquainted. Pay attention to what you do without thinking, how you feel, your tendencies and habits, what you like and dislike. It's not self-indulgent to spend your energy getting to know yourself. On the contrary, it's absolutely essential. Unless you really know yourself, you can't ever really know anyone else. And that's the heart of rule 8:

Know thyself.

This rule follows all the other rules around like a shadow, and makes them all work better. In fact, none of them will work very well without it, because a little self-knowledge helps make those rules work. So let's talk about you.

Who Are You?

Who do you think you are, anyway? You're not Oprah, Paris Hilton, Cameron Diaz, or Queen Latifah. Maybe you're built more like Beyoncé than like Nicole Richie, or you look more like Jennifer Lopez than Calista Flockhart, but you aren't any of those people, and that's good. You are unique and totally *you*. You aren't your sister or your mom or your best friend. So why do you keep comparing yourself to all those other people?

I strongly believe that it does not serve anyone to compare herself with anyone else. All that time and energy spent wishing you looked like, say, Victoria Beckham or Fergie would be much better spent getting to know *you*. You won't ever be anybody else. But you can continually improve on and better yourself. Isn't that what you should be thinking about? This is your journey with your own unique destination, and no one else's is identical.

You have a unique schedule, personality, metabolism, body type, lifestyle, and many other traits. Magazines and television brainwash us into having an unrealistic body image, to the point where we don't even realize what is actually attractive or what really looks good on *us*. Why would Jessica Simpson's ideal weight have anything to do with your ideal weight? For that matter, if you ask twenty men who attracts them, I guarantee you that many will choose Beyoncé, Jennifer Lopez, Fergie, Kim Kardashian, and Pamela Anderson over Nicole Richie, Lindsay Lohan, Calista Flockhart, and Mary Kate Olsen. Sure, they're all beautiful women, but many men like their women curvy.

But you aren't doing this for a man, either, right? Your first priority has to be *you*. When you concentrate on who you are and what you need, only then will you be able to be a good girlfriend, wife, mother, friend, and member of your community. All those roles are important, but they all start with you.

You can't be a size zero when you are six feet tall. If you are naturally a size zero, then that's fine. That's right for you. But if you aren't, forget about it. Why would you want to change who you are? You have to work with what you've got and find where your own beauty lies. Chances are, your beauty has nothing to do with finally being able to buy a pair of jeans with a two or four on the label. It will have more to do with you, looking *your* best, and playing your own game.

But how do you know what your game is? You have to start paying attention to *you*. This is when personal time becomes more than a luxury; it becomes a necessity. I'm not saying you shouldn't seek support from friends, because friends can bolster you, support you, and motivate you to be your very best self. But surround yourself with positive influences carrying you closer to your goals. Negative people can set you back. To be naturally thin, you have to be a little selfish, but the result will benefit everyone you know and love.

Knowing Your Own Hunger

Food is a great place to start gaining self-knowledge. One of the most important things to learn about yourself is what hunger is for you. Part of the problem I have with "eating every three hours" or "eating five times every day"—concepts often appearing in the media—is that not everyone is hungry so often; and even if you are this hungry on some days, you won't be on other days. Why eat when you aren't hungry? When each one of your days is different, doesn't it make sense that the way you eat will vary, too?

Or, maybe you are the kind of person who *does* have to eat when you aren't hungry because if you don't, you'll forget about eating until you are ravenous and then you won't be able to control yourself. This is exactly what I'm talking about when I say, ♡ *know thyself.* ♡ You might need to eat at certain times to keep yourself on track.

To keep your eating under control, you might need to eat three square meals every day and never snack. Or you might need to eat five times a day on some days, but only twice on other days. It all depends on you. It's futile and absurd for me to tell you that you have to eat only one way. I don't know what you like or how hungry you are right at this moment. I don't know what you had for breakfast or what you are going to have for dinner, whether you are going out to a restaurant or feel like cooking tonight. So how can I tell you when and how to eat?

But you know. You have to know yourself so that you can tell yourself.

This all dovetails with the notion that you are the one in control—not the food, and not any kind of diet. It's all about you, and you call the shots. Every day is new and different, and life changes, but you are always you and nobody knows you as well as *you* do.

I've always been a very independent person, and I like to feel I'm in control of my own life. I know a lot of other women who feel the same way. Why are these same women (myself included, until I snapped out of it) so willing to give up total control over the very intimate, personal, and influential act of eating? So, you're an amazing, powerful career woman with a great boyfriend or husband, a beautiful home, great kids or hobbies or passions or whatever, but when it's time for dinner you give up all your personal power to a cheeseburger and fries. You let a television commercial for a pizza run the show. Or you let a diet run your life and starve you until you're crazy.

Not anymore, you don't. Because by practicing rule 8, ♡ *know thyself,* ♡ you know yourself well enough to know that certain things set you off and you are going to avoid them. Other things make you feel great, so you will seek them out. You know how much of something is too much, and how much is just right for you. You don't look to a book to tell you to eat half a cup of pasta and a cup of vegetables when you'd rather have a grilled salmon filet, because you *know* what you'd rather have.

Knowing Your Triggers

Another, subtler part of really knowing yourself is knowing what makes you overeat—and what sets you off. What are your triggers? This is especially important if you tend to binge. For some of you, stress puts you in a position to overeat, but you will be a lot more likely to do it if you have sweets in the house. Others seek out crunchy, salty foods. If you have a weakness for pizza, candy bars, or nachos, you need to recognize this trigger food. Maybe you need to avoid it for a while, until you get better control of your situation and are planted firmly in the driver's seat. Or maybe you can begin immediately to see that trigger food in a whole new way, as something no longer forbidden. If you don't forbid it, you may not feel compelled to eat too much of it.

Do you see how it all depends on you? One person might not be able to keep chocolate in the house because she knows she can't possibly control how much chocolate she eats. Another might be able to keep it in the house with no problem because the simple recognition that chocolate is OK is enough to put the brakes on. Which one are you?

Skipping meals can also be a trigger for some people, but not for others. I do not agree with the idea that everybody should always stuff herself with food within five seconds of waking up. If I wake up and I'm not hungry yet, I won't eat right away, or I'll just have something small. I wait until I'm hungry to have a whole meal. However, not everybody can do this. For some people, breakfast, even when they aren't very hungry, is important to keep them from overeating later. Which one are you?

Just remember that skipping meals too often will eventually affect your metabolism. Most of the time, it is important to eat healthy meals. Just know that on some days, you might skip breakfast. You'll live. Or you'll know you should have a snack before you get too hungry.

Know thyself.

Writing Your Own Rules

Maybe you just need to think about who you are, where your strengths lie, what your food noise says, and how you like to eat. Or maybe you need to write it down. Writing down your own rules about how you like to eat can be a big help, but only if you see them as your personal preferences and qualities, rather than as self-imposed laws you are trying to enforce.

Think about you. Do you have predetermined dietary needs, like gluten or lactose intolerance? Do you choose not to eat meat? Do you choose to eat kosher? Do you prefer organic food, or raw food? Do you need meat to feel strong and healthy? These are part of your rules.

Your own personal rules might also have to do with your schedule. If you have to get to work early, you may prefer to eat breakfast a little later, once you are more awake and feeling hungry. Maybe you have a more flexible schedule and for you, it's very important to get up and relax over a nice breakfast. Maybe you don't do lunch but you always go out for dinner, or maybe you eat your main meal in the middle of the day and prefer to eat light at night.

Consider who you are, even if it feels selfish. Spend some time on this. Who do you want to be? How do you want to eat? How does eating fit into your life, and what are the best parts of your life that have nothing to do with food?

I'm not requiring you to write any of this down, but if it helps, please do that here. Sometimes, writing ideas down can clarify what you think, and that can take you a long way toward self-knowledge. I'll give you some space, along with some questions to think about, but if you want to keep going, please do. A self-knowledge journal? I think that's a great idea.

These are some of my favorite foods: _____
_____

These are the foods I really don't like: _____
_____

This is how I feel about breakfast: _____
_____

I have a hard time controlling my eating when I'm feeling: _____
_____

I do really well eating in these situations: _____
_____

I have a hard time limiting my portions when I eat: _____
_____

This is how I feel about eating out in restaurants: _____
_____

I would describe my food philosophy like this: _____
_____

I feel strong and healthy when I eat: _____
_____

Am I a grazer or a binger? I think that right now, my food personality tends to be: _____

_____

I'm really good at: _____

_____

I'm afraid of these foods: _____

_____

I would like to change these things about my eating: _____

_____

I believe I am naturally thin because: _____

_____

I'm also thinking about: _____

_____

_____

Be Prepared

As you continue to think about who you are and how you eat, also think about how you can best be prepared to meet the eating challenges you face in your everyday life. Everybody knows that being prepared can help you deal with the unexpected, but do you know how *you* need to be prepared? You can read and follow every hint, tip, and trick in all the diet books—stashing granola bars in your purse or whatever—but what if you don't like granola bars, or they put you into a sugar rut that you won't get out of all day? Being prepared is absolutely a good idea, but you have to ♡ *know thyself* ♡ to know exactly how to prepare for the kinds of situations you will face in your life.

HEAVY HABIT

Fasting is an ancient practice that people still apply today, for many reasons including weight loss and religious observance.

Fasting can be an effective way to flush excess water out of your system and make yourself feel thinner, but it can also be very challenging. I admit that I have practiced juice fasts in the past, drinking only freshly squeezed juice but not having any solid food for a few days. But the cleansing effects of fasting don't last, and fasting alone is not a good way to become naturally thin. A few people can kick-start a healthy eating regimen with a fast, but for many people, this backfires. ♡ *Know thyself.* ♡ If fasting is uncomfortable for you, don't do it.

But maybe you fast for other reasons, and fasting works for you. I'm not going to recommend it without the guidance of a doctor because it can be dangerous if you don't do it right, and telling you how to fast is beyond the scope of this book. But I will say this: some people can fast, and some people can't. If fasting is torture for you and you end up eating much more after you are done than you would have eaten if you hadn't fasted, this difficult practice is not for you. If you can do it safely and in a healthy way, then that is up to you. But you really have to know yourself (and talk to your doctor) before you decide to try fasting. (Stay tuned for my book on cleansing!)

As with everything in life, being prepared with food choices makes us more efficient and successful. Camping without a tent and a plan isn't wise, nor is launching a new eating lifestyle without any tools for making it work. If you want to eat to be naturally thin, you have to be prepared and ♡ *know thyself* ♡ at the same time.

Let me give you some examples. Let's say you work in an office and you're constantly surrounded by junk food. Fast-food restaurants are everywhere and everybody is always asking, "Do you want me to bring you back anything?" If that's tempting to you when you get hungry, you'd better have emergency healthy snacks and prepacked lunches with you each day. The few minutes it takes to bring healthy food choices with you may be all it takes to help you just say no to junk food.

But suppose you know you are the kind of person who, even though she has an apple and a turkey sandwich in her purse, is likely to say, "Oh, all right, you talked me into it. Bring me back a double cheeseburger and a large order of fries." Then, it won't do any good to pack healthy snacks. You have to up the ante and either bring something better that you know you really want to eat, or figure out how to order from restaurants in a healthy way. If you, personally, need fast food now and then, fine. Have a small hamburger, a small order of fries, and a bottle of water. Or skip the fries and get a small shake. Or get cheese on the burger but forget about the fries or the shake and get a side salad. Be smart, and pick what *you* really want most. Remember, ♡ *you can have it all, just not all at once.* ♡

If you're faced with convenience store food, know that more and more of these stores now have fruit, cheese, sandwiches on whole-grain bread, and other healthy choices. But if you must have a candy bar or some chips, read the labels and make the best pos- sible choice—candy bars with nuts or baked chips made from soy or whole grains with less fat are smarter investments than a lot of other choices. If a label has more than five ingredients or you don't recog- nize what the ingredients are, I advise finding something else. And don't forget the water. Staying well hydrated when you are running around all day will really help you feel better and help calm your hunger so you can make a wiser investment.

The point is to have a strategy for all the situations that normally pop up in *your* life. Maybe you work at home. Do you get up and raid the refrigerator every time your work starts to get tedious or you aren't sure what to do next? If that's you, then ♡ *know thyself.* ♡ You won't be a person who can keep junk food in the house. Freeze more fattening foods so they are harder to access, and put the fresh healthy foods in the front of the refrigerator or cabinet. Have a few quick, easy, healthy recipes on hand that you can make in less than five minutes, or put together homemade food into sensible portions in plastic containers so your lunch is ready to go and you have no excuse not to make a smart investment.

I can't map this out for you, because I don't know what your days will be like and what challenges you face. But you can sit down and think about this, plan ahead, and be ready. Think about what, in your normal life, you need to do for breakfast, lunch, snacks, and dinner, and make sure you have what you need. This is all part of your commitment to yourself—to being naturally thin. A few minutes spent in preparation will pay off a hundredfold when you find yourself in a situation where you are tempted to make a bad investment.

Preparation Ideas

I provide custom meals for my clients at work, so I know how easy this can be if you simply take the time. Purchase reusable plastic containers, and either prepare every day for the day ahead or—even better—prepare several days at once. Buy your supplies at the grocery store, then spend an hour preparing meals and snacks for the next few days. This is an hour invested in a valuable commodity: your own good health. This is also a great way to use leftovers when you've cooked a big dinner, or when you've brought home a lot of extra food from a restaurant.

Here's how I do it:

- Line the bottom of containers with different types of salad greens. Top them with your favorite protein—it could be canned tuna, chicken from the night before, sliced leftover steak, or baked tofu. Then add a sprinkling of some flavor such as cheese or nuts, and combine with colorful veggies such as tomatoes and bell peppers. Fill a small plastic container with a low-fat packaged dressing to go with it. Add a slice of whole-grain bread, some brown rice, or whole-grain pretzels or something else crunchy and starchy. Voilà, you have a light, healthy lunch you can take with you or keep easily accessible at home.

- Another good meal to make ahead and store for a convenient lunch or dinner: soup. Especially in the winter, a pint of nice homemade soup will do wonders for your waistline, as well as for your attitude. On one night, sauté onions, carrots, and celery; add your favorite chopped vegetable with salt and pepper and a container of chicken stock. Puree, season to taste, then separate into several containers for high-volume snacks or lunch sides. Some canned soups are great, too. I love Amy's soups. Some boxed soups are also very good and low in calories but high in flavor. Read the label.

- For healthy morning and afternoon snacks, keep small containers of Greek yogurt in the fridge with individually portioned plastic containers or snack bags of low-fat granola or fruit and nuts. Another easy snack: whole wheat pita wedges with store-bought hummus or a slice of whole-grain bread with low-fat cheese or peanut butter. Whole-grain pretzels with a slice of cheese would be a great afternoon snack, too. If you have healthful foods you actually like in the refrigerator, you'll grab them.

- Edamame is a delicious and protein-rich snack.

- The cucumber salad recipe in Chapter 7 is a great one to make and save when between-meal hunger hits you.

- If it's sweets you crave, then make up portion-controlled containers of dark chocolate and almonds (the healthy fat in the almonds helps to balance the sugar in the chocolate) or combine whipped cottage cheese, honey, maple syrup (or Splenda), vanilla extract, and chocolate chips (or make my faux cheesecake recipe on page 41). This can be made in several variations, such as with slivered almonds and almond extract. Divide between small containers for something quick, sweet, and delicious.

The possibilities are nearly endless, but the point is to make up the snacks in portion-controlled batches *before* you get hungry—and to make snacks that *you will actually eat.* Don't fool yourself into thinking that if you have no food, you won't eat. When the body is hungry, it finds a way to eat. Whether you will be going to work, to a gym, on a road trip, or to an airport, be ready for hunger. When you make meals and snacks yourself, they will taste better and be better for you than processed junk food. Desperation usually results in poor choices.

Once you understand and adopt this concept and it becomes second nature, you might wonder why you never practiced it before. Why wouldn't you eat really good food you made yourself? Why wouldn't you order food that will make you feel good, not sluggish and bloated? But the only way to make these new practices into habits is to make them fit you and your life. Let self-knowledge be your quest.

Rule 8 Recipes

These recipes make small, delicious snacks that are just right for spoiling your appetite so you can make better investments throughout the day, especially before a big food-centric event. Make them ahead and store them for easy access. You'll feel better, calmer, and more prepared knowing that you've got homemade food to eat instead of packaged junk. (You'll save money, too.)

Pomegranate Smoothie

This smoothie is simple, quick, and so refreshing. When you aren't that hungry for breakfast in the morning, try this recipe. I think it's perfect without the additional sweetener, although some people like their smoothies sweeter, so go with your own preference—but try it without sweetening first, just to see if you like it.

Serves 2

1 cup berries (such as raspberries, strawberries, or blueberries)
¼ cup pomegranate juice

¼ cup water

½ banana

1 cup ice

Optional: A little bit of Stevia, maple syrup, or honey, if you want it sweeter

Combine all the ingredients in a blender and blend until smooth. Enjoy!

Butternut Squash Puree

I want to let you in on a little secret, one of my all-time favorite quick snacks. I'm not a huge snacker, but this is such a great snack in the middle of the day.

1 serving

Buy a box of frozen butternut squash at the store. These little boxes (I buy the ones by Cascadian Farms but Birdseye also makes it) have the squash all prepared for you, so you don't have to peel and chop it. Microwave it according to the directions, then mash it up with just a dab of butter and some cinnamon, or simply salt and pepper. This is incredibly delicious and so easy, and the calorie count is low. I eat this all the time.

Chapter 9

GET REAL

As you've probably noticed, I have a problem with processed food. I think a huge part of America's obesity epidemic, not to mention our emotional slavery to food, is directly related to processed food, which is fast and easy to make, quick to consume, full of artificial ingredients, and ultimately unsatisfying. I'm not a scientist, but from my experience and from what I read, chemicals in food can have a big impact on our physical life as well as our emotional life, contributing to mood swings, sugar highs and lows, irritability, and depression.

That brings us to rule 9, a rule close to my heart and in my opinion, one solution for getting all of us back on track to eating the way our bodies are designed to eat:

Get real.

In other words, *eat real food.*

Unfortunately for us, the world is now filled with fake food. The makers cheerfully advertise that it will make us thin and healthy. But I say: if a food comes in a package, you generally want to avoid it. Once again, this is a more European mentality, where processed food is much less accepted and pervasive. Of course there are exceptions, but if you start paying attention to how processed your food is and how different processed food tastes compared with real food, you will see why this is so important. I want you to start getting picky about the food you eat, so that you gradually train your palate and your body to recognize and appreciate real food. Plus, packaged food costs a lot more. A simple bag of rice is, for example, a whole lot cheaper than a packaged "rice dinner," if you break it down per serving.

What Is Real?

What is real food? Ask a dozen people, and they will probably have a dozen opinions about where to draw the line. But the way I see it, in our current society, food exists on a spectrum, from totally natural (you just pulled a carrot out of the garden) to totally fake (do you recognize even half the ingredients on the label of that energy bar or "meal-replacement" shake?). Fruits, vegetables, whole grains, organic dairy products, organic chicken, and wild-caught fish are all real foods. Packaged foods are less real.

I want you to keep your eye on the real end of the spectrum.

Real food doesn't come in a package. It doesn't have a label. And it's obvious, when you look at it, what it is: a banana, a chicken, a freshly baked loaf of bread. Real foods include fresh vegetables and fruits, whole grains, organic beef, chicken, pork, and fish. But of course, "real" isn't always simple. Is milk from a factory-farmed, hormone-infused cow a "real" food? Is it better than a carton of soy-milk? What about a package of plain frozen, microwavable broccoli?

Is that worse than a mayo-drenched bacon-filled broccoli salad at a potluck dinner?

What is real or what is a good investment isn't always a matter of black or white, because some processed foods can actually be good investments—some of the time. There is plenty of room for choosing the better versions of packaged foods—unsweetened shredded wheat cereal, corn chips with oil and salt and nothing else, Bethenny-Bakes vegan cupcakes.

There are also plenty of easy ways to *get real* without being obsessive. You are trying to live without thinking about food all the time, so I don't want you worrying about this too much. If you get so worried about making sure every bite is 100 percent real and natural, you'll drive yourself crazy. This is not a rule of extremes, so let's make it easy.

First, choose food as close to its natural state as possible in your current situation. An apple is better than pasteurized apple juice, but apple juice is better than "apple-flavored drink" that doesn't contain any apples or contains, say, only ten percent real juice.

A fresh salad full of raw organic vegetables is better than canned mixed vegetables that you heat up on the stove, but a can of organic vegetables is better than a frozen microwaveable plastic tray of tasteless vegetables drowned in salty sauce full of chemical preservatives.

When you have a choice, pick what is most natural, assuming it looks good and it is what you want. Do the best you can. That's what I mean by *get real.*

One reason I believe it is so important to eat real food is that your body understands real food. The body knows what to do with it, how to digest it, how to use it. If you throw diet sodas and microwavable sludge at your body all day, you are probably not going to be as healthy or feel as good. It may sound trite, and you've heard it before, but you are what you eat. What you eat also affects how you look—your hair, your skin, even your expression.

Almost Real

But let's be honest here. I eat processed food sometimes. I might be traveling and have no choice but to get food from a convenience store or a fast-food restaurant. I don't like it, but it happens. And I do actually enjoy some processed food. I complain about those energy bars, but I enjoy a good veggie burger now and then, and those burgers are highly processed, even if they are a smart investment in other ways. It's a case of the lesser of evils.

Honestly, I even make packaged food through my company, but my BethennyBakes vegan muffins, cookies, and cupcakes are made with healthy natural ingredients you can pronounce and contain no animal products. They are a great investment when you want something sweet and you don't want to go overboard. But they are processed.

Sometimes, your only choices, or even your best choices, will be processed foods. You should know that some are better than others so choose the lesser of evils. For example, if you have to have fast food, a veggie burger is a better choice than a double bacon cheeseburger. A veggie burger has less fat, more fiber, and fewer calories, and in my opinion, it tastes better. I know I feel better after eating it than I would after eating a huge fat-filled burger. (But remember, if you like fatty burgers, they aren't forbidden—just have only a few bites, and a high-quality burger in a nice restaurant is not the same as a fast-food burger.) Choose a lower-fat or peanut-filled candy bar over straight chocolate or something without any protein. Choose soy crisps, whole-grain chips, or crackers and cheese over a big bag of greasy potato chips.

But choose what you *like*. Remember the *differential*. Choose the best thing for you that will actually satisfy you, then stop when you've had enough. Use common sense, too. A veggie burger dripping with oil on a white bun? Not necessarily a good choice. Just be mindful. *Pay attention,* and you'll know what choice to make.

Get Picky

If you are really committed to being naturally thin, you need to become more discerning about what you decide is worth putting into your mouth. Care about how your food tastes (first, of course, you have to ♡ *pay attention* ♡ to how it tastes). Care about what you are putting into your body, and how it will affect you later. The simple fact is that in most cases, fresh, real, organic food tastes better.

When you choose to eat more real food, you'll refine your palate, learning to appreciate what tastes good and what tastes fake. You'll also begin to notice how food affects you. Maybe you can't get your rings off before you go to bed because your fingers are swollen, or you wake up the next morning and your ankles look like an elephant's ankles. These are signs your body is sending you that whatever you ate did not sit well with you. And chances are that this food was processed, full of salt and chemicals. You won't feel swollen after eating real food.

But I also know that if you are in the *habit* of eating mostly processed foods, it's hard to stop. That stuff is addictive: it's a vicious cycle. It's so easy that you hardly have to worry about dinner. If you usually take five minutes to make your dinner and five minutes to eat it, I know perfectly well that you aren't going to transform yourself overnight into a gourmet cook who spends hours each day shopping at the market and slow-cooking a healthy meal.

If you've been living on processed food, it may take you a while to appreciate the taste of fresh fruits and vegetables, organic chicken, free-range eggs, and whole grains. But believe me, they will win you over if you give them a chance. You'll feel so much better that you won't ever want to go back to junk food. Let's take a closer look at why it's worth switching back to real food, and how you can do it in real life in a way that works for you, without changing your entire lifestyle.

CELEBRITY SECRETS

When Denis Leary was filming his television show *Rescue Me,* I cooked for him on the set, in his trailer, using a small oven and a tiny microwave (it wasn't easy cooking for six of his cast members on this minimalist equipment). Denis was a tough case. He was a real junk-food eater. He would live on cheeseburgers and chicken Parmesan. He hardly ever ate anything green.

Then I started making fresh delicious food for him, and healthy alternatives to his favorite junk food, and guess what. He didn't even notice. But he did notice how much more energy he had, and how good he started to look. He's learned to love broccoli rabe, arugula, and baked chicken wings, in addition to the cheeseburgers and fried chicken he likes.

But Denis hasn't given up his favorite foods. He still indulges. The difference is that he's learned to love his healthy choices, and he feels great, even though he still occasionally eats junk food. If Denis Leary can learn to love healthy food, so can you.

Go Organic When You Can

One of the first, relatively easy steps in nudging your diet toward the more real end of the spectrum is to go organic. I don't mean for everything, all the time, every bite. Not everybody can afford to buy everything organic, and not everybody has access to organic food all the time, either. But when you have a choice, it's worthwhile to try organic food.

Organic foods have multiple benefits that more than make up for their higher cost, even if you eat only a bit of organic food:

- Organic foods don't have pesticides or other chemical residues on them.

- Organic foods are grown in a more earth-friendly way, without chemical runoff.
- Organic foods are grown in a more humane way. Animals can't be cruelly confined or mistreated, and must be fed an organic diet themselves.
- Organic foods may contain more nutrients. Without the aid of pesticides, organic plants have to fend for themselves and have been shown to generate more antioxidants and other natural substances that can benefit you when you eat them.
- Organic foods taste better.

It's easier than ever before to choose organic foods. Even stores like Wal-Mart and Costco carry organic food now, and because larger companies have realized that organic food sells, they are getting involved. But don't forget the farmers' market, where family farmers—many of whom can't afford to be certified—are nevertheless producing food without pesticides and other chemicals.

I don't buy everything organic, but I am more likely to choose organic food when it matters most. For example, fruits and vegetables with very porous, thin skins will absorb the most pesticides. Strawberries, spinach, and grapes are very susceptible to pesticides. A fruit with a thicker skin such as an orange, lemon, or banana has a protective outer layer, so arguably it is more difficult for pesticides to penetrate. Mushrooms should be organic, since they should never be rinsed, only wiped off before cooking.

Go Seasonal When You Can

Also, choose food that is in season, when you have the option. Seasonal food is not only fresher and tastier but a lot less expensive. In December a grapefruit costs half of what it costs in July. In July a peach is at its perfect ripeness, but a peach shipped from a foreign country in the middle of winter will be not only pricier but dry and flavorless.

Nothing is more flavorful, nutritious, and satisfying than fresh-picked corn, tomatoes, artichokes, and asparagus in the summertime. That is why during the winter, it is often better to use canned or jarred tomatoes. In winter, the tomatoes in supermarkets are mushy and inferior, whereas the canned ones were picked and packaged at their peak. Not only is this way of eating and thinking more healthy; it is more cost-effective and more satisfying.

You can learn a lot about what is in season each month by visiting your local farmers' market. In the spring, you'll be offered baby peas, radishes, and new greens. In the summer, you'll see tomatoes, peppers, eggplants, peaches, and berries. Come fall, you'll get apples, pears, walnuts, pumpkins, and butternut squash. At a farmers' market, you can often browse food that has been picked the same day. It's hard to get fresher and more seasonal than this.

Learn what foods come into season when, and plan your eating around nature's calendar.

NATURALLY THIN THOUGHT

When drinking fresh squeezed juices, please drink organic. When I do a juice fast, I always drink organic. Otherwise I feel as if I'm injecting pesticides directly into my body.

Go Local When You Can

Whenever possible, choose local food. I live in New York. Why would I choose an apple from New Zealand when I could choose an apple from upstate New York that didn't have to travel so far, is fresher, and is less likely to be doused in chemicals and waxes in order to make a long trip? Sure, sometimes the New Zealand apple is the only choice, and it will taste perfectly good. But if you have a choice, get your food from local sources.

Eating locally goes hand in hand with eating seasonally, so once again I will encourage you to visit your farmers' market, or the produce stands that farmers set up on roadsides in the country and in small towns. No food can be at its optimum flavor and nutritional value when it has been shipped thousands of miles, has been ripened in a box (often by gassing), and finally gets to you weeks after being picked. Eating a mango from Costa Rica isn't as wise a choice as eating a beautiful peach during the summer on the east coast. Now, I don't want you to feel intimated, either. This is a goal, not a rule. Nine times out of ten, I shop at the supermarket. I eat mangoes in the winter. But I shoot for going as real as I can, when it works in my life. This is not something to stress about!

But if you do have some good local markets, enjoy them! Eating local isn't limited to vegetables and fruit. Some farmers' markets sell fresh local chicken, lamb, pork, or beef; and depending on where you live, you might even be able to get fresh local seafood, artisanal cheese, and local olive oil. You can also get freshly baked local bread, special-occasion desserts, and dinner from a tamale stand or an outdoor barbecue. When you get used to shopping and eating like this, the grocery store will begin to seem cold, sterile, and unappetizing.

Eating locally and seasonally helps the environment, too. You'll be voting with your dollars to reduce agricultural chemicals in our water, reduce the fuel needed to ship food long distances, and support the small family farmer. If you can be naturally thin while also helping to keep beautiful small farms from being replaced by shopping centers, McMansions, or huge industrial factory farms, then you can feel good about yourself in more ways than one.

Variety Is the Spice of Life

Very often, I go shopping for food with friends and clients and discover that they always buy exactly the same things. They eat the same meals every week; they are stuck in a food rut. Either they stick with what they like, or they think their families won't want to try new things. I understand that people know what they know, and are sometimes intimidated by change. I see the same reaction when people order in restaurants. They know they like something, so they order it all the time. Maybe this sounds corny, but I truly believe that variety is the spice of life.

Nowhere else can you find nature's amazing variety like in the world of real food. Take some time, walk down the produce aisle, and see what looks vibrant and interesting. You'll start to notice how some of the choices change as the seasons change, while others are always there (shipped from other countries). Notice which things look good, fresh, and ripe at which times, and try to pick what looks best *today*, rather than always getting what you always get, whether it looks good or not.

Some people are afraid to try a new vegetable or a new fruit because they don't know how to cook it. But the truth is that no vegetable takes very long to prepare in a simple, delicious way. Do you always make the same salad? Do you buy the same greens, vegetables, and dressing because they are safe and you know you like them? Small changes make a world of difference. I cook for clients every day, and surprise them with the smallest alterations, with big results.

Add new vegetables to your salads, like sweet grape tomatoes, grated red cabbage, crunchy diced celery, fresh chives, baby peas or corn kernels, and roasted vegetables like eggplant, mushrooms, and

---

NATURALLY THIN THOUGHT

Even when you think you have no food in your house, I bet you can make a salad. Sometimes just having herbs or sugar snap peas is enough if you add a dash of olive oil and some lemon juice. I made a salad of celery, tomatoes, baby carrots, red onions, and cilantro. That was all I had in the house, along with bleu cheese dressing. It was a meal. You can make a salad out of almost any vegetables.

---

bell peppers. Break out of your vegetable rut by sautéing or roasting broccoli or spinach with garlic and olive oil, squeezing with lemon, and sprinkling with Parmesan. Marinate portobello mushrooms in a store-bought balsamic vinaigrette and broil them in the oven or grill them on the barbecue.

For a main course, a simple piece of fish, chicken, or meat can be made many different ways with small changes in herbs, spices, and oils. Even side dishes can be made more interesting with micro-adjustments in seasoning. When I cook for clients, one day I might mix brown rice with olive oil, salt, pepper, and mixed chopped herbs. The next day, I might simply bake a sweet potato, then top it with maple syrup, cinnamon, and olive oil. Whole-grain pasta can be changed in shape and by substituting simple ingredients. One day, combine the pasta with shredded basil, sun-dried tomatoes, and feta cheese. The next day, use low-fat ricotta, olive oil, garlic, sautéed spinach, and a sprinkle of Parmesan. Then, when you are feeling lazy, mix the pasta with store-bought pesto and finish with lemon zest, a few pine nuts, and a sprinkle of Parmesan cheese.

You might notice that I repeat certain basic flavoring ingredients a lot. My basics are olive oil, fresh garlic, lemon, salt, and pepper. Very often, I'll use freshly squeezed lemon juice or zest, or both. As for "accessories," my staples are packaged pesto; sun-dried tomatoes; pear tomatoes; spinach (fresh or frozen, but drain the frozen kind); Parmesan, feta, or goat cheese; basil; parsley; dill; and cilantro. By mixing and matching these flavors, you can go from French to Mediterranean to Mexican in moments, and you'll never wish your food had more flavor.

Eat the Rainbow

I often tell my clients to eat the rainbow. In other words, look for color in your food. The more colors on your plate, the better. This rule is a great rule for you, and it is also fun to pass on to your children. Basically, real foods that are naturally bright in color have the highest nutritional value. Foods such as pomegranates, sweet potatoes, spinach, arugula, tomatoes, berries, broccoli, kale, and many more are the ones that are filled with antioxidants.

You know perfectly well I'm not talking about artificial colors here. No, a strawberry margarita doesn't count. (Unless it's made with fresh organic local strawberries, in which case it's actually better. Studies show that a little alcohol could make the antioxidants in fruit more available to the body.) But strawberries, blackberries, blueberries, and watermelon—yes! Generally speaking, if it is a whole, natural food and it could stain your clothing, it is probably good for you.

CELEBRITY SECRETS

Years ago, I was a personal assistant to Jerry Bruckheimer, producer of films like *The Rock*, *Pearl Harbor*, and *Armageddon*. For me, Jerry and his family really embody rule 9. Not only are they real, genuine people, but everything in the Bruckheimer home is organic, natural, and fresh. Jerry is as precise about what he eats as he is about the movies he produces.

Eating the rainbow doesn't mean that vegetables such as cauliflower, iceberg lettuce, or white potatoes are bad for you. In fact, they are healthy, high-fiber foods with their own set of benefits. However, if given the choice between iceberg and romaine, go for the romaine because of its darker color. Going further, choose arugula or spinach over romaine, for the same reason. All things being equal, a sweet potato is a better choice than a baked white potato. Brown rice is better than white rice. Dark whole-grain breads are better than breads lighter in color.

This rule holds true for fruits as well—that is why blueberries, goji berries, cranberries, and pomegranates are called superfoods. They are nutrient-dense. I'm sure there are some exceptions, but as a rule of thumb, eat foods that are bright in color and loaded with nutrition and you'll get even more power out of rule 9.

Turn Up the Volume

Another very important reason why eating real food can help you become naturally thin is that real food is, in many cases, high-volume food. Raw vegetables, in particular, are high in fiber and volume, so when you eat them *first,* you end up with less room in your stomach for other, higher-calorie food. Start your meal with a big salad or a bowl of vegetable soup, and you won't have much room left for food with more fat and calories. If you start your meal eating a piece of white bread from the breadbasket or a sugary doughnut, you are left as hungry as before.

Other real food is high-volume, too—brown rice, whole-grain pasta, bran cereal, fruit, soup, and beans all help you to feel full and satisfied. Those are wise investments.

HEAVY HABIT

Volume eating is great, but like anything else, it requires some common sense. Eat an apple, but not three apples. Eat a mango, but not ten. Eating fruit alone on an empty stomach can be cleansing, but the natural sugars can cause your blood sugar to spike and crash, leaving you hungry. Instead, when you eat fruit (as you should do at least once a day), try to eat it with a small amount of protein to offset the sugar. Eat an apple with some nuts or peanut butter. If you don't manage to eat protein with your fruit, you aren't going to die, but it's a goal. Combine berries or melons with Greek yogurt. Spread a little soft cheese on your pear slices.

I always think about volume when choosing foods. Look at one serving of whole-grain pretzels, and you'll see that the calories are similar those in a serving of potato chips, but look at what each food weighs. I guarantee you that for the same number of calories, the whole-grain pretzels will occupy more space in your stomach, leaving you more satisfied. You'll get to eat more, for the same calorie expenditure.

Focus on volume for your side dishes, too. Instead of french fries, opt for a small baked potato, beans, or squash. Substitute whole-grain pasta for white pasta if possible; and when ordering pasta, choose a dish with a variety of vegetables. If you eat the vegetables first, you will eat less of the more caloric pasta. Do the same with pizzas. If you crave pizza, choose a slice topped with high-volume vegetables. This way, one piece will satisfy you, and maybe you will leave some of the crust. Have a salad first, and you'll eat even less.

When you are making hamburgers, steak, chicken, or fish, try to incorporate vegetables into recipes and sauces when possible, so you will fill yourself on low-calorie, high-volume food. Adding a few leaves of lettuce and a slice of tomato will increase the low-calorie volume of a burger. Onions and peppers can go into chili, zucchini or pumpkin into dessert or breakfast bread, and soup is the perfect palette for high-volume vegetables.

Once you get used to eating real food, you'll wonder how you could ever have stomached all that processed fake food, and this will be an important step in your progress toward becoming naturally thin. Sure, you'll always have your favorite junk food. I do, too. But if it becomes a "I know what this is going to do to me, so I'll have only two bites"—kind of thing, then you'll be eating like a thin person.

Rule 9 Recipes

These recipes all use fresh seasonal real food in a beautiful palette of colors. They are also high-volume, so you'll fill up and feel satisfied on fewer calories.

These salads, featured last year in the culinary issue of *Hamptons Magazine* in an article I wrote about upscale, healthy barbecue, are great to make for a party. Displayed together, they make an impressive and artistic presentation. Or make just one of them for a beautiful lunch. Color means not only that the food is more nutritious, but also that it looks much better. I'll buy the yellow tomatoes in addition to red just to have more colors.

Each salad serves about 4 as a meal, or 8 as an appetizer. (Of course, you can always make half or a quarter of these recipes, to serve fewer people.)

Rainbow Salad

8 cups baby spinach, well washed

1 cup quartered grape tomatoes

1 cup thinly sliced orange bell peppers

1 cup baby corn, raw or grilled

1 cup halved sugar snap peas or chopped asparagus (quickly steam them first, then dip them into an ice bath to preserve the color)

1 cup shredded red cabbage

1 cup chopped hearts of palm

Salt and pepper, to taste

1 cup chiffonade of fresh basil (finely sliced basil leaves)

½ cup low-fat ranch dressing and ½ cup light vinaigrette dressing mixed together

1. Arrange the baby spinach on a platter. Over the spinach, make rows out of each of the vegetables: a row of tomatoes, then a row of peppers, then a row of corn, etc. Season the salad with salt and pepper, to taste.

2. Sprinkle the entire salad with the chiffonade of basil. Combine the ranch and vinaigrette dressings, then drizzle them evenly over the top of the salad.

Tomato Mozzarella Salad

With red and yellow tomatoes and green and purple basil, this salad is even more spectacular.

Serves 6

2 fresh ripe red tomatoes

2 fresh ripe yellow tomatoes

1 pound fresh buffalo mozzarella in water (Costco has a great brand)

½ cup fresh basil leaves

Salt and pepper, to taste

¼ cup fresh green pesto (can be store bought)

1. Core the tomatoes, then cut into ½-inch slices. Slice the mozzarella so you have half as many slices of cheese as tomato slices.

2. In one or two rows (depending on the size of your plate or serving platter), layer the tomatoes and cheese, alternating a slice of red tomato, a slice of cheese, and a slice of yellow tomato.

3. Arrange the basil leaves over the tomatoes and cheese. Season with salt and pepper, then drizzle the entire salad with pesto.

Pureed Vegetable Soup

Something about pureed food feels nurturing to me. I love this delicious soup, not only because it represents comfort to me but because it always makes me feel clean and energized after I eat it, especially when I use real fresh seasonal vegetables. This recipe is versatile. You can use any vegetables that are in season and look particularly good, or you can make it to use up leftover vegetables you happen to have sitting around, while they are still fresh. Freeze the leftovers in small individual containers so you always have some pureed vegetable soup whenever you need it.

Serves 4

1 medium red onion, chopped
Nonstick cooking spray
6 cups chicken or vegetable stock or broth
½ cup chopped celery
½ cup chopped carrot
2 cups chopped asparagus, broccoli, cauliflower, or a combination
Salt and pepper, to taste
Juice of ½ a lemon
Your favorite fresh herbs, for garnish

1. Over high heat sauté the onions in a large pot, using the nonstick cooking spray, until slightly soft. Add the chicken or vegetable stock or broth, all the vegetables, salt, and pepper. Simmer until the vegetables are soft.

2. Turn off the heat. Using a hand (immersion) blender, puree the mixture until smooth. Add the lemon juice. Season with more salt and pepper, to taste. Garnish with your favorite fresh chopped herbs.

Chapter 10

GOOD FOR YOU

This is the last chapter in Part One, and the last rule. It's also an important rule that wraps up all the other rules, and it's about *you*. But this chapter goes beyond ♡ *know thyself.* ♡ Without this chapter, the other rules would be hollow and meaningless, because this chapter underpins each of them. Rule 10 wants you to do what is:

♡ good for you. ♡

I talk a lot in this book about how I am not going to tell you what to eat or how much, when to exercise or in what way, or how to live your life. That's because what you do, and who you are, is your choice. It's your body, and your *life*. I want to empower you to take control of who you are and how you want to live, including what you want to eat, how you want to feel, and how you look. But I also want you to take care of yourself, and that's this rule's focus.

My role is to show you how to be *you*—but you as a naturally thin person, because being thin *is* a part of who you are, even if you don't see it today. It can be a part of who anybody is, if people will only let themselves be thin.

Are You Allowing Yourself to Be Naturally Thin?

This is an important part of rule 10: *let yourself be thin*. Being overweight isn't good for you, nor is being obsessive but being naturally thin—whatever naturally thin is, for you and your body—*is ♡ good for you. ♡* To get there, though, you need to let yourself be thin. Are you doing that?

I'm serious. You might think, "Of course I want to be thin!" But think about it. A lot of people have a lot of food noise that gets in the way, telling them that they won't ever be thin or that they are more comfortable or more protected if they have an extra layer of fat. Are you letting your weight protect you? Are you afraid to look good? Are you afraid it will be too hard? Are you afraid of giving up your best excuse for why something isn't working in your life?

Well, you need to cut that out. Change can be uncomfortable at first, but I am here by your side as you do this. A lot of people are very afraid of a little discomfort, and I understand that, but the reward is so big that paying closer attention to how you eat and taking control of how you live are well worth the initial and temporary inconvenience of changing a few bad habits.

When you change for the better, you will learn that the discomfort will quickly be replaced by a feeling of rightness, and of getting back into your own skin, where you belong. Don't be fooled by clever, devious food noise that tells you it can't happen to you, or even that you aren't ready for it to happen, or that you don't deserve it. That's a big fat lie. Remember, food isn't your best friend, and it isn't your enemy. It's just food. It's no big deal. *You* are the big deal, and you deserve to be healthy, strong, and thin. But I can't do it for you, and nobody else can, either, despite what people might tell you on the covers of their books. Only you can let it happen.

Sometimes, just realizing that you are sabotaging yourself is all you need to do to stop. But sometimes it takes longer. Some habits are hard to break, and it can take some time. But that's OK. Start paying attention to why you overeat and when, how you feel when you are tempted to make a bad food investment, and what benefits being overweight has for you. This is all deeply rooted in conscious-ness- in simply waking up. ♡ *Pay attention* ♡ to what you do and think and feel every day of your life.

Yes, for some people, being overweight really does have (seem-ing) benefits, as I mentioned before: safety, protection, and a great excuse. An excuse for what? For not being in a good relationship? For not having a great job? For not putting on a bikini and risking uncomfortable exposure? For being able to blame your parents for your life, since you inherited their weight problems and so it's all their fault?

That's crap. You don't have to wear a bikini. Plenty of naturally thin people don't. And frankly, the extra layer of fat is not protecting you in any real or useful way. Your life is your own, and shifting the blame for it onto anybody or anything else is just an excuse not to live it. I understand why you might think that way, believe me. I've been there. But the simple truth is that your relationships, your job, your comfort level with your body, and your parental issues are all things that thin people struggle with, too.

Getting thin is not going to solve all the problems in your life, and if you think it will, you are sorely mistaken. But getting thin can do something else even more important: it can set you on the path to-ward *caring* about yourself. Once you do that, you'll be able to tackle those other problems a lot more effectively. Do this first, and you'll get off the wrong path and set your feet firmly on the right one.

Thinking that a weight problem is causing other problems in your life is in itself an excuse. If you aren't really ready to get into or out of a relationship, you might be telling yourself that you have to figure this out first. Then you'll be able to lose weight. Or you have to resolve things with your parents, or get a better job. I'm not saying that you shouldn't try to do those things, but you have to separate them from *this* thing: getting naturally thin. Let yourself let go of the weight you are carrying around like a burden. When you decide to put it down and walk away from it, it will go away. Let this be a separate issue—a matter of doing what's best for you.

HEAVY HABIT

Stop waiting around to fix everything else in your life before you start taking care of yourself. If you aren't fixing those things now, what makes you think you're going to start anytime soon? Take care of yourself first, and the other things will fall into place.

Exercise

Here's a fact: I don't exercise as much as I used to. I rarely have time to get to a gym. But I am very active. I'm always moving, not sitting on a couch. It's more of a European mentality.

So I'm not going to be hypocritical and tell you to go to a gym every day. Some people just don't have the time or the desire to do that. I used to take a spin class every day, but now my life feels like a spin class and I don't have time to add any more spinning! I actually wouldn't mind going to the gym more often, but I just don't have the time.

Some people hate gyms. I understand that. No problem. Nobody is telling you that you have to go to a gym. People don't exercise in Europe the way they do here in America, and I think that's significant. They walk everywhere, they are active, they climb stairs, and they spend time outside, but they think it's weird to "work out" every day. Yet they are thinner than we are.

Obviously, exercise is good for you, but my point is that exercise comes in many forms. Pick what works for you, what you enjoy, and what you will actually *do*, even if that's just going for a walk every day, walking to work, taking a yoga class, or working in the garden. Or just try some gentle stretching. If you like going to the gym—I know a lot of people who do—then great, do that. Exercise calms you and quiets your food noise.

But over-exercising can actually be counterproductive. It can give you a raging appetite; it can result in injuries such as stress fractures; and it can become an obsession, setting you on a figurative treadmill where you exercise, overeat, exercise, overeat. You have to find a balance in your life. Don't let exercise—or food—rule your life, but incorporate both into your life in a calm way, with you in the driver's seat.

That being said, do something. Get outside. Breathe. Move. It's *good for you.* Here are some ideas to inspire you:

- **Try yoga.** There are many types of yoga, from gentle stretching meditative forms to more active forms that raise a sweat. Talk to yoga teachers near you to find a style you like, if yoga appeals to you. Some yoga centers offer classes in a variety of styles. If yoga isn't your thing, that's fine, too. I love yoga, but not everybody does. However, give yoga a chance. Try it three to five times before you decide you don't like it.
- **Walk.** Humans are built to walk, not to sit in desk chairs all day. Walking is free, it's relaxing, and you can walk fast or slowly depending on your fitness level and how you feel on any given day. Walk every day, and it will get to be easier and more fun. If you get to that level and your body is built for it, you can even start running, but you can get a really good workout just by walking, so don't pressure yourself.
- **Ride your bike.** Why drive when you can ride and not have to fill up the gas tank? Riding a bike is not only more economical and eco-friendly, but also a great exercise—and it puts you out there in the world in a much more interesting way than staying safely sealed inside your car. (But wear a helmet and follow the rules of the road!)

- **Swim.** If you have a pool nearby and you love the water, try swimming a few times a week. Swimming is great exercise that puts no stress on your joints. Some people don't like it, but for others, there is no better exercise. Try it and see which type you are.

- **The gym isn't so bad.** Some people love going to a gym, where they can be around other like-minded exercisers. These days, gyms usually have many options. For inspiration, you can take exercise classes, from easy to challenging. You can get on a stationary bike and take a spin class, or you can relax or get sweaty in a yoga class. You can lift weights—this is great for your muscle tone and will increase your body's ability to burn calories. Or you can just pop in, do the treadmill or elliptical trainer for thirty or forty-five minutes, and go home without ever talking to anybody. Some gyms also have pools where you can swim peaceful laps at your own pace. My gym has a steam room, and I consider a steam my reward for exercising. At a gym, you can exercise no matter what the weather is like. Look for specials to attract new members, and you can probably joint at a bargain price. Some companies have special deals with gyms or even offer corporate reimbursement. If you hate going to a gym, fine. But if you try it, you might find out that it's fun.

- **Play sports.** Some people would rather play a game than "exercise." Sports are great exercise, though, so if you can find one you like, go for it! Get moving by playing tennis or racquetball, taking a ballet class, skiing or water skiing, snowboarding, ice skating, or joining a local league that plays soccer, baseball, football, or whatever.

My point is that because exercise is ♡ *good for you,* ♡ you should do something. But don't force yourself to do something you hate, or you won't keep it up. Start slowly, move gently, and let your body adjust. Work it into your schedule in a realistic way. I only get a chance to exercise about two or three times a week, but even that makes a difference. Find exercise that feels more like fun than like work, even if it's just walking or biking to and from your job. Pretty soon, you'll be hooked—and feeling and looking great.

Sleep

Most of us don't get enough sleep, and that's a serious problem. Sleep deprivation can suppress your immune system, allowing you to get sick more easily. It gives you brain fog, so you can't concentrate or perform as well at work, at school, or even in a conversation. Children who don't get enough sleep can have behavioral problems, and adults who don't get enough sleep feel tired all day. For some people, that results in not only excessive caffeine consumption but excessive appetite. Studies have shown that people who are sleep-deprived eat more, especially more starchy foods like pasta, bread, and sugar.

According to the National Sleep Foundation's annual survey for 2008, sixty-five percent of respondents reported sleep problems at least a few nights a week, and nearly half said they woke up feeling unrefreshed at least a few times a week. On average, people said they needed a little more than seven hours a night to function at their best, but most don't usually get to sleep that long. Also, those who were considered obese were more likely to sleep less than six hours a week on workdays, and to drive while tired.

In other words, sleeping matters, and sleep is *good for you.* Sure, you can sleep too much, and that's not good for you, either. But if you are one of those people who just don't have time to sleep enough, or who are in the habit of staying up too late and then regretting it in the morning, I suggest taking a serious look at your sleep habits.

You will have an easier time feeling calm, eating less, being less hungry, and controlling your decisions about food if you are well rested. So turn of the television and go to bed. Let sleep be a higher priority, and you'll be doing something very good for you and your body. Here are some tips to help you get a better night's sleep:

- **Turn off the television.** That noise, those flickering lights, and that electricity are not conducive to restful sleep. If you are in the habit of falling asleep with the television on, it's worth trying to go without, at least a few nights per week. Your sleep will be sounder and more refreshing.
- **Indulge in comfortable, luxurious linens.**
- **Clean up.** If your bedroom is clean, you might sleep more peacefully. Clutter in a room can make you feel stressed and anxious. When the space around you is clean, calm, and serene, you'll feel that way, too.
- **Ritualize.** Studies show that if you have a nighttime ritual, you will fall asleep more easily. Whether it's taking a bath, reading a book, drinking a cup of noncaffeinated herbal tea, or listening to music, do that one thing before bed every night and your body will know exactly where it's going.
- **No caffeine after 3 p.m.**
- **Turn in early—sometimes.** If you are chronically sleep-deprived, try setting aside one night per week (even if it is difficult to do it on the same night each week) to turn in early, relax, and catch up. If you get only five or six hours a night, a solid ten-hour sleep one night per week might be just what you are craving.
- **Stretching.**
- **Meditate.** Meditation techniques teach you to calm your anxious, racing thoughts so you can finally drift off. Teaching you how to meditate is beyond the scope of this book, but look into meditation if you think you could benefit. It's like yoga for your brain, and you'll think more clearly during the day, too.

Bottom line: Let yourself sleep. Sleep is very important, and it will make everything in your life work better.

Participate

One of the many reasons I object to dieting is that it keeps you from participating in your life. You always worry that the restaurant your friends want to go to won't have anything you can order, or that your host at a dinner party will serve fattening food and you might have to turn down something and risk being rude. You worry about vacations and dates. You even worry about how to cook something at home so it will fit into your diet.

I don't want you to worry. I want you to participate in life. Why should you have to be sidelined, just because you are trying to lose a few pounds? It's ridiculous. Live! Go out with your friends, go on dates, go on a vacation, and *enjoy yourself.* Food is only a small part of those experiences anyway, so focus on the other wonderful aspects of living and socializing, like talking with your friends, getting to know new people, and exploring interesting new places.

Participating is also ♡ *good for you* ♡ because it helps build your confidence and self-esteem. Of course you are going to go to that party. Of course you are going on that date. Of course you will participate in the girls' night out. When you participate, you stop feeling as if something is wrong with you. Follow the ten rules as you go, and you'll feel even better as you get naturally thinner.

NATURALLY THIN THOUGHT

If you follow the ten rules, you'll be able to participate in anything life throws at you without fear that you are breaking your diet. That's the beauty of being naturally thin. It's about living, not about dieting. It's about participating, not waiting to participate until you have achieved some number on a scale. It's about not being obsessed with food so you can finally enjoy food.

Love Yourself

It's easy for me to say, "Love yourself," but it wasn't so easy for me to do. I had a tough childhood, so I know what it's like to feel bad about yourself, even to punish yourself by overeating, yo-yo dieting, or starving yourself. But after a lot of work, I rose up out of that. If I can do it, you can, too.

How can you not love yourself, when you are all you know? You have ultimate access because you are inside your own head and you can make yourself into the best possible version of yourself. But you have to care about yourself, take care of yourself, and love yourself, by doing what is truly ♡ *good for you.* ♡

It's great to have friends, a family, a life partner who care about you—sure. But none of that is going to work very well if you don't care about yourself first. Put yourself and your own needs ahead of everything else, and you'll begin to see why this is the only way you can then turn around and be a good friend, a good family member, a good parent, a good partner. Loving yourself has to be at the very heart of everything you do.

This is really hard for some people because they are so used to putting themselves last. But that's not going to get you anything other than feeling miserable and feeling bad. Then you compensate by developing unhealthy habits like overeating or substance abuse.

It may take a while, but start doing little things for yourself every day. Always give yourself at least fifteen uninterrupted minutes of "you time." Do little things for yourself throughout the day: have a piece of fruit; go for a walk; take a break from your work to breathe deeply; eat a square of dark chocolate; or just sit in a hammock. Give someone a hug. Hold your boyfriend's hand. All these little things will help you learn how to take care of yourself, and care grows into love.

Do you see why you need to do what's ♡ *good for you* ♡ before you can ever make the changes necessary to become naturally thin? In some ways, you could argue that this should be rule 1, but I have learned that it works better to ease into this rule. Not everybody is ready to hear it at first.

Nevertheless, doing what is ♡ *good for you* ♡ really does work together with all the other rules, and is an important part of getting naturally thin in a sound, healthy, permanent way. You get one life. You deserve to make it the best it can be, so figure out what you need, what you want, and who you want to be.

Then be.

Rule 10 Recipes

These recipes are just for you—special treats that still won't break your nutritional bank. Indulge yourself, but use these recipes to do it wisely.

Rustic Mashed Potatoes

What embodies comfort food more than any other dish? To me, it's mashed potatoes. This version includes the skins, for extra nutrients. Creamy white beans add texture and protein.

Serves 4 (If you are cooking for one, portion out the rest into freezer containers so you have mashed potatoes ready for any time you crave comfort.)

4 medium russet potatoes, well washed
One 12-ounce can white beans, drained
½ cup warm plain soymilk
⅓ cup ricotta cheese
¼ cup butter
1 tablespoon salt
Dash of pepper

1. Cube the potatoes but leave the skins on. Put them in a pot and cover with water. Cover the pot and bring the potatoes to a boil. Cook for 25 minutes, or until very tender.

2. Meanwhile, puree the white beans in a food processor until smooth. Drain the potatoes. Put them back in the pot, add the bean puree, and add the remaining ingredients. Mash everything together. Heat through and serve hot.

Citrus Shrimp Refresher

This light, cleansing, elegant appetizer feels luxurious. On a light-eating day, paired with a salad, this can be dinner.

Serves 1 (Double it if you are making a special dinner for 2.)

2 large shrimps, split in half, tails removed
¼ of a cucumber, peeled and chopped
¼ of a segmented pink grapefruit
¼ of a segmented lime
1 teaspoon fresh cilantro, minced
¼ of an avocado, cubed

Combine all ingredients in a small bowl, then serve in a chilled cocktail martini glass.

SkinnyGirl Frangelini

This Frangelico-flavored martini is delicious and tastes decadent, but has virtually no sugar and very few calories compared with most fancy sweetened martinis. To order it, just ask for vanilla-flavored vodka on the rocks with club soda, with just a tiny splash of Frangelico. Or make it at home.

Serves 1 (You can increase it easily for larger groups, making several glasses at once.)

1 shot of vanilla-flavored vodka (count 1, 2)
Club soda
Splash of Frangelico

Fill a rocks glass with ice. Add the vodka, then fill the glass with club soda. Add a splash of Frangelico on top. Cheers!

Part Two

THE NATURALLY
THIN PROGRAM

Chapter 11

THE NATURALLY THIN
PROGRAM: SETTING IT UP

Now that you have a good knowledge of the ten principles of eating and living naturally thin, it's time to put those principles into practice. To help you do this, I'm going to walk you through a week, helping you to make the ten principles a real part of your life. I'll also provide you with the details of what I'm eating in a typical week, with some thoughts about why I'm making these choices. Give me seven days, and I'll give you the greatest gift I know. I'll show you exactly how to be naturally thin.

Maybe you weren't naturally thin yesterday. But that was yesterday. Today—the day you begin the Naturally Thin Program—and for the next seven days, put your trust in me and you will begin to understand exactly what I mean when I talk about living, thinking, and eating like a naturally thin person. Remember, *this is not a diet because diets don't work*. This works because this is your life.

The Naturally Thin Program is different from a diet. With the ten rules you've already learned in Part One of this book, along with your own willingness to get rid of the heavy habits that have been weighing you down, you can finally uncover the naturally thin body you always knew was yours. It's going to be fun, and it's going to be easier than you think, because this doesn't involve deprivation. It's a program of balanced decision making—because ♡*your diet is a bank account.*♡

Time to Quit Dieting

The first week of the program is extremely important because if you haven't already given up dieting for good the moment you read Chapter 1, this is the week to do it. This is the week when you *quit dieting*. You're going to banish the whole notion from your head, forever. Once, the idea of dieting was ingrained in me, too, so I know that the idea of quitting sounds a little scary. Now, however, I never diet, I never obsess, and I never fear any food. I never will again. There is no tomorrow; there is only right now. If I'm hungry, I eat. If I'm not hungry, I don't eat. And when I'm not eating, I live my life. This is what I want for you.

It sounds simple, but it can take some practice, and that's where the Naturally Thin Program kicks in—to help you practice listening to your food voice, shutting out your food noise, and eating when and what you really want, not what or when a clock, a diet plan, or someone sitting next to you in a restaurant says you should eat.

Why do I include the Naturally Thin Program in this book, if I'm so opposed to diets? Isn't the point to teach you how to do this yourself? Exactly. For some people, the ten rules alone aren't enough structure, so for those of you who want more structure, here it is. I can talk all day about how I think, how naturally thin people think, and how you can change the way you think. But when you are faced with a restaurant menu, a bakery case full of cupcakes, or a hot cheesy pizza at midnight, you're going to need something to hang on to. That's what this program is all about. This is me, holding your hand and walking through the week with you, to show you how it works to live and eat this way.

But what the Naturally Thin Program is *not* about is me telling you to eat half a cup of this and three tablespoons of that. I'm not going to do that, because that goes against everything being naturally thin is about. Humans are strange creatures, and every one of us is different. This morning, I had a small vegan coconut cupcake and half a cantaloupe for breakfast. How could I possibly put that on a meal plan for you? Maybe you hate coconut, or cantaloupe. And it certainly wasn't the breakfast of champions!

But I will tell you what I am eating, because I want you to hear my inner dialogue when I decide what to eat. If you do like the sound of it, you can get inspiration from my meals. You can also get an idea of portion control and the way I balance the foods I eat throughout the day. However, my meals aren't meant to be a meal plan for you. They are meant to be only a tool to help guide you through your own meals. I want to empower you to make your own decisions about food. Only then will you be in the driver's seat. Naturally thin people don't eat what other people tell them to eat. They eat what they want to eat, and what their bodies need and want. No more, and no less.

The good news is that nothing is off-limits. *Nothing.* And nothing will ever be off-limits again. No restaurant, snack, drink, lack of exercise, or personal choice is "bad." It's how your choices string together that determines your weight, your energy level, and how you look in your jeans. Think of it this way. You might snap at somebody in a rash moment. You can then decide you are a snappish person and keep on snapping, or you can apologize (or not) and get back to being the person you know you are. It's the same way with food. You make decisions, one at a time, and then you make more decisions based on the ones you've already made. If you mess up, you make it right with your next decision. *You* are the one in control and the one who will deal with the consequences of your decisions. You are the *only one* who can change your weight and your life.

But I can help you.

I'm with You

My challenge, in developing the Naturally Thin Program, is that I don't believe in rigidity, strict portions, measuring food, or counting calories. It's just not practical. It doesn't work. You might do it for a few days, but then you're going to throw your measuring cup into the sink and start eating out of the box. It's too frustrating, because it's not how people really live.

The other challenge is that people are not stamped out with cookie cutters. I've had couples ask me if I could put them both on a diet program, but the truth is, when you, your husband, and your kids or you and your friends sit down to the same meal, you don't all suddenly become the same person. Add to this the simple fact that when you sit down to lunch today, you and your day will be a little different from what they will be tomorrow. You and your friends and family members each have different backgrounds, schedules, metabolisms, and styles. You have different activity levels and different favorite foods. This makes each of you unique, and also makes it absolutely absurd to pick up a diet book and strictly follow a regimen somebody else designed.

You can't please everybody and you certainly can't magically dissolve everybody's weight problems with such a diet. It's not possible. I'm not even going to try.

Instead, what I'll do here is walk you through each day, implementing the ten naturally thin rules and applying those to *whatever foods you like to eat*. This works, and it works fast. But you aren't changing who you are. You are just tweaking your bad habits and turning them into good strategies—naturally thin thoughts and actions.

Move through the week and these chapters as if I'm hanging out with you, telling you what I'm eating and helping you apply the rules to what you are eating. You won't be eating the same things I'm eating, because we aren't in the same situation and we have different preferences. Maybe one night you'll be going out and I'll be eating in, or I'll be going out and you'll be eating in—or whatever. Either way, I'll be with you, as if we'll be going out for dinner together, but we won't have to order the same thing.

The point is that no matter where you eat and how your day is going, you won't be eating alone. I'm right here, working with you and discussing all the different issues that come up. I'll also keep reminding you of the ten rules, until they are ingrained in your life and have become your new habits. The same rules apply to both of us, and we'll both be eating the naturally thin way, so it will be a journey we take together.

Trusting Your Food Voice

In Part One of this book, I talked about food noise. I believe many of us have a lot of food noise in our heads. It's an obsessive voice that tells us we can't eat this, we must never eat that, we can't possibly touch even a bite of something else. Then it turns on us and commands us to eat everything in sight because we feel deprived or stressed out and we "deserve" to eat. But then it makes us feel guilty about what we did, and subsequently tells us we don't deserve anything good again. Or it tells us how good and virtuous we are when we don't eat.

Sometimes my food noise tells me to eat too much sugar. Yours might tell you to eat half of a pizza, instead of the one piece you had planned on. You can't trust food noise, because it is deeply rooted in negative emotions: self-disparagement, anxiety, stress, and heavy habits. I'm here to help you identify and ignore food noise.

What you *can* trust is your *food voice*. To review, your food voice is a deep inner wisdom that tells you when you are hungry, when you really aren't hungry, and what you really *want* to eat.

Listening to your food voice—your inner voice—teaches you how to communicate with yourself. It's that simple. When you learn to listen to your food voice, you will begin to understand that it's perfectly fine to have a fried egg and a piece of bacon or a small piece of chocolate cake or whatever you really want. You don't have to finish it all (since you've ♡ *canceled your membership in the Clean Plate Club* ♡). But you get to eat what you really want—for the rest of your life.

The Rules

Part One deals in detail with ten rules you can follow to finally achieve natural thinness. I want you to memorize and live by these rules, so let's review them briefly here:

1. ♡ Your Diet Is a Bank Account. ♡

This most important rule is the guiding principle behind the Naturally Thin Program. No matter what you decide to eat, base your choices on balancing throughout the day, so you don't eat too much of any one thing and each meal balances the others with complementary food choices.

2. ♡ You Can Have It All, Just Not All at Once. ♡

Life is about choices. You can eat whatever you want, and you should eat a variety of things to make food as interesting and nutritious as possible; but at the same time, you need to keep it simple. Fill up on high-volume, healthful foods like salads and soups; then pick the one or two things you really want. Have the salad, the pizza, and the wine. Or have the soup, the salad, and the dessert. Remember, you'll always have another chance to make a different choice. You've got plenty of meals in your future. Make your choice and go with it.

3. ♡ Taste Everything, Eat Nothing. ♡

Why shove a bunch of food into your face when you can taste small perfect bites of delicious food and stop before it ever gets ugly?

Be choosy and discerning, especially when you have a lot of great choices. If you can't decide, have just a taste of everything you really want, and you'll still respect yourself in the morning.

4. ♥ Pay Attention. ♥

Never eat until you are ready to pay attention to what you are doing. Don't eat while standing up, working, driving, or watching television. Sit down, experience your food, and savor it so your body registers the meal.

5. ♥ Downsize Now! ♥

Forget supersizing. Downsizing is your new way of life. Eat from smaller plates, bowls, and glasses, and cultivate a new sense of portions.

6. ♥ Cancel Your Membership in the Clean Plate Club. ♥

Quit finishing everything on your plate. The fact that it's there doesn't mean you have to eat it. Instead, share your food, save it for another meal, or just leave it when it really isn't very good.

7. ♥ Check Yourself before You Wreck Yourself. ♥

This rule encompasses one of the most important things you can do for yourself: *stop binge-eating.* Never do it again. Just knowing you can have any food you want can keep you from going overboard, but until you break the binge habit, you need to stay firmly in the driver's seat and make your own rational decisions about what you will and will not eat, and when you will stop eating it. You are the master of your own life, so step up.

8. ♡Know Thyself. ♡

Some people can skip meals and some can't. Some people have a weakness for sugar, and some can take it or leave it. Some people can eat a little pasta, and some can't. Some people need snacks, and some don't. Are you a vegan? Gluten-intolerant? An exercise fanatic? As you reframe your habits, you have to know yourself and customize the way you eat to fit who you are.

9. ♡Get Real. ♡

Whenever possible, when you have the option, without getting obsessive about it, choose real, organic, local, seasonal food instead of fake processed food. Sometimes processed food is the only choice, but when you can choose to eat fresh fruits, vegetables, whole grains, or organic proteins, go for them. Your body and the earth will thank you.

10. ♡Good for You. ♡

Every habit you change should come from a gentle place of caring for and loving yourself. No matter what you decide to do, how you decide to eat, and who you decide to be, let yourself be guided by what is ♡ *good for you,* ♡ ahead of anything else. Do this, and everything else in your life will fall into place.

The Differential and the Point of Diminishing Returns

As long as we are having a quick refresher course here, let's talk about two key concepts that I explained in Part One, and that I really want you to remember: the *differential* and the *point of diminishing returns*.

The *differential* is the difference between two choices, and whether or not that difference is worthwhile. If the healthier version of a food is pretty much just as good, in your opinion, go for that choice. If the more decadent choice is *way worth it,* then go for the splurge. (But have just a little. There's no need to hurt yourself.)

The *point of diminishing returns* is the point after which a food doesn't taste quite as good. The first few bites of any good food are full of flavor and excitement. But as soon as the excitement starts to wane—as soon as a bite you take is a bit less great than the bite you took before—you might as well stop. Cut your losses and put down your fork.

Balancing Basics

Now let's talk about how to incorporate these ten rules and other concepts into your life, when you are going to work or school or restaurants, when you are faced with feeding a family or shopping at the grocery store or going out with your friends. Remember the first rule: *Your diet is a bank account.*

But how can you do it? To help you, I'll give you some basic guidelines about how to balance your choices. These are just guidelines. I don't want you to obsess or go crazy over this. What your food voice tells you is the most important thing. Learn to listen to your body.

I want to emphasize that on your most hungry days, you might eat a little more than what I offer as a guideline. On other days, you will eat less. Never feel that you have to spend everything in your bank account. If you aren't hungry, why stuff yourself? That's just being mean to your body. Yes, there will be days when for some reason—or for no reason—you are starving all day. But on days when you aren't starving, save. I don't eat breakfast every day. So sue me. I'm thin, and I eat when I need to eat. Sometimes I include breakfast, and once in a while I don't. But I'm not saying that's right for you. Each day is different, and eating something just because you are supposed to have *x* number of servings of whatever is absurd.

In general, however, *on those days when you need some direction,* here's what I'd like to see you striving for, in order to balance your diet like a bank account.

> One or two meals based on carbs preferably whole-grain or vegetable rather than refined as in whole-flour or white pasta

Every day, one of your meals can be all about carbs, pasta, rice, a sandwich, pancakes, or whatever. This doesn't mean you won't eat some protein, too, and vegetables are always good to add, but when the focus of the meal is carbs, count that as a carb meal. Besides, you don't need to clog up your digestion with too many different kinds of food at one meal.

I'm not going to list every kind of carbohydrate-rich substance on the planet, because you aren't stupid. I'm not going to insult your intelligence by telling you exactly what a serving is in ridiculous detail, either. I don't want you to obsess. You can go back to Chapter 5 for more specific information about serving sizes if you want to, but you know perfectly well how much is too much for you. A carb meal might include one or two carb servings. As a brief reminder, here are some generalizations about serving sizes for carb foods:

- Bread, 1 slice (half a slice if it's a huge or thick slice; whole-grain if possible)
- Whole-wheat or whole-grain bagels (I scoop mine, which means I pull out the extra bread and throw it away, because I like bagels better that way). Get the small ones, not the ones the size of your head.
- Muffins the size of a small apple (whole-grain, if available). I'm not going to tell you how many ounces—you know the difference between a big muffin and a small muffin. If you can find only a big muffin, cut it in half. Otherwise, it counts as two servings.

- Whole-grain cereal, small cereal bowl or Japanese rice bowl, about the size of half a grapefruit
- Whole-grain pasta, small bowl (as above)
- Rice, small bowl (as above), preferably brown or wild rice
- Corn, ramekin
- Potatoes, sweet potatoes, winter squash (butternut, acorn, etc.) small bowl (or half a large baked potato)
- Beans and peas, like black beans, white beans, chickpeas, black-eyed peas, etc.

> One or two meals based on protein, preferably lower in fat

Every day, one of your meals should focus on protein, to help balance the carb meal. This meal may also contain some carbs, but protein will be the focus. For example, scrambled eggs with half a toasted pita is a protein meal. Have the pita, toast, or whatever, but make it a small serving. Protein is important and keeps you full longer than starchy foods, but you can certainly overdo it. One or two meals featuring lean protein each day are plenty. If you have eggs for breakfast and steak for dinner, you don't need meat for lunch. As for the leanness, if you are really dying for protein that is higher in fat, like a prime rib or a hot dog, that's fine every now and then. Just don't eat the whole thing. Most of the time, choose small portions of lean protein, such as:

- Fish (salmon, tuna, etc.), shrimp, or crab, a serving about the size of a small sponge
- Chicken, a smaller portion if you like dark meat or the skin (as I do), a slightly larger portion if you like the skinless boneless breast
- Beef. I like the fatty pieces, so I eat less. If you like the leaner pieces, such as a plain fillet (without the extra pat of butter restaurants often add), you can have a bit more.
- Low-fat cottage cheese with a small handful of nuts

- Eggs. Have one egg if you have other protein, like bacon; have two eggs if they're your main protein source. If you eat the yolks, skip the cheese. If you prefer cheese on your eggs, try using egg whites only. Remember: balance.
- Tofu, firm or extra-firm, about the size of a small sponge. I prefer the low-fat variety because of the *differential*.
- Beans (black, white, pinto, garbanzo, etc.). Serve them in a small bowl or ramekin. They are high in protein but starchy, so they really straddle two categories.
- Low-fat cheese or soy cheese or both, 1 slice or a small handful. If you prefer full-fat cheese, have just a sprinkle.
- Skim or low-fat soymilk, about one cup

> 2 fruits (including juice), and unlimited vegetables
> (except starchy veggies)

Fruit is a great investment, but too much fruit will make your blood sugar spike. Alone, fruit is cleansing and has a lot of important nutrients, but remember that it isn't filling for more than a few minutes. It's great for dehydration and recovery when you aren't feeling great, but be smart about it. In general, stick to two fruit servings a day, including fresh juice. One of these might be part of a meal, such as fruit with breakfast. The other could be a snack. When it comes to veggies, eat as much as you want (except potatoes and corn, which count as carbs). Raw veggies are especially important. This is where you can really fill up. Focus the bulk of your diet here. Vegetables make you feel good and full. You can do thousands of things in the kitchen with vegetables (many of the recipes throughout this book show you how), and this category has lots of filling, regulating fiber. When you learn to choose really good, ripe, seasonal fruits and veggies and prepare them the right way, you'll learn to love them, and you'll be wondering how you ever lived without them as the centerpiece of your plate.

2 fats

Have a little butter or olive oil twice during the day. These fats add a lot of great flavor, but you don't need much, and you certainly don't need to put them on everything you eat. Don't douse everything with fat, but don't banish fat from your life, either. Fat is not the devil. It's actually good for you in small amounts.

Fat can come in some obvious places, like bacon and eggs, and some less obvious places, too, like sautéed vegetables. If you order sautéed vegetables in a restaurant, don't think you aren't getting any fat. But don't skip the vegetables for this reason or replace them with some other, less healthful source of fat. I don't know anybody who ever got fat eating too many sautéed vegetables. In general, you won't really need to think about adding fat to your day because chances are good that the foods you choose will contain enough fat, or you'll use it in cooking.

Honestly, when I go out to a steakhouse, for example, I probably eat more than two things with fat. Don't freak out about this or obsess about "two servings" of fat. That's not what I mean. I just mean that fatty food should be part of only two of your meals.

2 sweets

If you love sweets as I do, you know it can be hard to be sensible. Have no more than two small sweets every day, including breakfast, snacks, desserts, and sweet after-dinner drinks. If you have sugar on your oatmeal and a cookie in the afternoon, that's it. No ice cream after dinner. If you want the ice cream, skip the cookie or don't put sugar in your coffee. Balance your sweets. You don't *need* more than two, so pick the ones you want most. If you don't care much about sweets, then have a sweet just once, or not at all. Sweets are not a dietary requirement. Alcohol counts as a sweet! If you have two glasses of wine, that's your sweets quota for the day.

OK, I admit I often have more than two sweets in a day, including the days when I have a few drinks. I'm maintaining now. Be more careful if you want to lose weight, but don't get too stressed if you go over once in a while. Nobody is going to send you to food jail.

2 snacks

These should be pretty small. Aim for approximately 100 to 200 calories for a snack, but don't obsess about the number; this is just a ballpark figure. Snacks also have to be balanced with your meals, so I usually recommend that one snack is more on the sweet side (that counts as one of your two sweets), and one is more on the salty side. Choose your snack on the basis of the meal you had before it, and don't follow bread with bread or protein with protein. Balance is the key. A small snack of starchy food or protein doesn't have to count as one of your two servings. I'm not going to tell you what you have to eat for a snack, but I'll tell you some of my faves:

- 1 slice of Ezekiel sprouted-grain bread with a slice of soy cheese and a slice of tomato
- 1 large spoonful of hummus and 1 handful of toasted pita chips
- Small glass of juice diluted 1:1 with mineral water
- ¼ bar of dark chocolate, with almonds to balance the sugar
- 1 piece of a decadent cupcake or brownie, when I'm really craving sugar (you know—PMS)
- A small salad lightly sprinkled with nuts or cheese, even if I'm not sure I'm in the mood for one. It fills me up and I'm always glad I had it afterward. You can never get too many fresh vegetables.
- Edamame
- Amy's organic soups. This company makes delicious soup. Soup is a great snack because it's filling, and soups full of veggies and beans are high in fiber.
- Gazpacho is a great snack.

- Fruit with a few nuts
- Small bag of soy crisps
- BethennyBakes cookie, muffin, or cupcake (you can find these at www.bethennybakes.com)
- Small low-calorie smoothie. Jamba Juice makes good mango and strawberry low-calorie smoothies.
- 1 Boca burger (or your favorite brand of veggie burger) on 1 slice of sprouted-grain bread, with or without 1 slice of soy cheese

The bottom line is that snacking spoils your appetite, and that's just what you want to do. A snack with 150 to 225 calories before an event will save you hundreds of calories at a party or restaurant meal.

2 beverages plus 6 to 8 glasses of water

If you want to drink alcohol, go ahead, but try to limit yourself to two drinks a day, and always have a glass of water between drinks. Sometimes I have more—this is just a guide. Remember, every alcohol drink counts as one of your sweets. If you have two drinks, then try to nix the sugar for the day, or only have a few bites of something sweet. That will count as an "exception." (See the next section.)

Always choose clear liquor over brown, and don't add sugary mixers. You can make a wine spritzer by adding seltzer to wine. (For more on drinking alcohol, see Chapter 16.)

As for other beverages, choose them wisely. I don't think anybody should ever drink soda. This is a place where I have trouble saying that if you like it, have just a little. It's just fake: high-fructose corn syrup or artificial sweetener with artificial flavors and colors. It's disgusting and addictive. I don't count it when I say that no food is off-limits, because soda isn't even a food. It's really not something anyone should be drinking. I'd much rather see you drinking sparkling water with a splash of real juice.

Diet drinks not only taste fake but, even if you get used to them and grow to like the taste, they are not good for you. They put you on a path toward sweet foods. Recent studies suggest that artificial sweeteners confuse the bodily chemical signals that tell you when you are full. You don't need something else whispering in your ear to confuse your food voice, especially now that you are trying so hard to listen. But I cannot tell a lie. I do use artificial sweetener sometimes. I don't drink diet soda, but when I have a cup of coffee, sometimes I put artificial sweetener in it. Sometimes I put it on cereal, too. So don't think I'm so perfect and telling you what to do. I'm just giving you an ideal. In any case, I strongly suggest you banish soda from your life.

As for other beverages, stick mostly to water, flavored with lemon or lime if you like. If you drink enough water that you aren't dehydrated, you'll be less likely to confuse thirst for hunger. Sometimes I crave juice, so I'll mix a little with seltzer or have just a few sips. Juicy fruits are obviously a better investment because they contain some fiber. Sometimes a slice of watermelon or a grapefruit will quench your thirst better than any sweetened beverage could. My favorite thirst-quenching beverage is Synergy brand Kombucha tea. I'll talk more about that in Chapter 13.

2 Exceptions

Every day, you can make two exceptions, if the opportunity arises and you think it's really worthwhile. Exceptions might include:

- 2 bites of a really great dessert
- 2 bites of an overly rich entrée like lasagna or fried food like calamari or fries
- ½ a piece of really good bread with a little olive oil or butter
- 1 small glass of wine or a few sips of an after-dinner drink

Here is a summarized version of the Daily Naturally Thin Program Account Balancing Guidelines. Remember, you don't have to eat everything on this list every day. Your life won't always work out that way. This is simply a guideline to help you with balancing your account.

Every day, balance your account by including approximately:

- 1 carb-based meal
- 1 protein-based meal
- 1 carb- or protein-based meal (or a meal with a balance of each)
- 1 sweet snack (under 225 calories)
- 1 savory snack (under 225 calories)

Also aim for:

- 1 or 2 fruits (if having two fruits, one should be a snack)
- Unlimited vegetables
- A total of two sweets throughout the day, including your sweet snack (which could be fruit), any alcohol you drink, or any desserts you decide to have
- Two exceptions—two or three bites or sips of something really decadent

That's it! Simple, right?

Remember, every day is different and you what you eat won't always fall in line with these guidelines. They are *guidelines*, not rules, and not a diet. This is something to aim for, especially if you are a person who needs more structure.

The following chart shows you how you might combine these basics over the course of three days, and how they can vary quite a bit from day to day. The chart includes possible protein and carb meals plus snacks, since those are the areas that give most people the most trouble.

You will probably get all the fats you need in your meals, so don't worry about adding those. Same with fruits and vegetables—eat those (especially vegetables) whenever you get the chance and remember to fill up on a salad before eating the more caloric parts of your meal.

This chart is not a meal plan for you, it is just an example of how to balance your choices like a bank account as you learn the naturally thin language. Once you've got it down, you'll be off book in no time.

THREE DAYS OF EATING FOLLOWING THE NATURALLY THIN PROGRAM:

DAY:	BREAKFAST	LUNCH	SNACK	DINNER	DESSERT/ SNACK
MONDAY	*Carb meal:* Cereal with fruit and soymilk	*Protein meal:* Grilled chicken salad with a sprinkle of nuts or cheese and a light vinaigrette	*Sweet snack:* Bethenny-Bakes cupcake	*Protein meal:* Sushi rolls (6 pieces) and sashimi (a few pieces) with edamame and a salad *Sweet:* Glass of Chardonnay	*Savory snack:* Small handful of cocktail nuts
TUESDAY	*Protein meal:* Vegetable frittata with feta and half a toasted pita	*Carb meal:* Bruschetta appetizer topped with tomato and mozzarella salad	*Savory snack:* Bag of soy crisps	*Carb meal:* Vegetable stir-fry over brown rice, soup	*Sweet snack:* Fruit skewers with a few nuts
WEDNESDAY	*Carb meal:* Toasted whole-wheat scooped bagel with soy cheese and a light spread of butter	*Protein meal:* Tuna and mayo over greens with a few whole-grain crackers	*Sweet snack:* Small scoop of all-natural low-fat ice cream	*Protein meal:* Linguine with clams, eating all the clams and just a little linguine	*Savory snack:* Small bowl of popcorn

At the end of this book, you'll also find a chart that shows what I ate over a three-week period. In that chart, after each meal, I'll note how I've balanced my protein, carbs, and sweets—since those are the main culprits in overeating for most people. You'll see that I don't always meet the Naturally Thin Program guidelines, but on most days, I come pretty close. I don't think about it anymore because it is habit. In the same way, I don't want you to get obsessive about this. Remember, this is just a general guideline for you to follow until you've learned the language and are eating to be naturally thin without giving it a second thought.

Following this method gives you the freedom to quit fearing food right now. You can quit weighing and measuring everything. And you can quit dieting. It's time to unshackle yourself and start living.

Putting the Rules into Practice

Now that you have the rules, the tools, and a basic sense of how to balance your food choices during the day, let's walk through the week together. I'm doing this with you, and you'll be able to see how I apply the ten rules and the Naturally Thin Program to my own life, as well as how you can apply it to yours. At each meal, I'll talk about different choices you can make, the choices I tend to make, and how it all works together and stays in balance.

I'll give you lots of examples of what you might choose to eat, with ideas for increasing the worth of your investments through the concept of the *differential* (like choosing whole grain over refined grain, adding fruit or vegetables, or making substitutions), for those times when you think the healthier choice is just as satisfying. Remember, this is about eating what you really love, as well as what makes you feel great.

Looking at what I do in my life can help you to understand how you can follow the Naturally Thin Program no matter what situations arise—whether you are at an airport, working overtime, on the run, eating out, or spending a day at home. This program gives you power over unusual circumstances. Today I had to film a segment for the *Today* show. Tomorrow I'm on a plane. Next week? Who knows. Life *is* an unusual circumstance. That's why diets don't work.

Let me be your guide and I'll hold a megaphone up to your food voice. If you focus on these rules and follow the Naturally Thin Program for seven days, you'll feel like a different person—lighter, calmer, more in control of your life, and *thinner*. As if you were born that way (and by the way, you were).

Chapter 12

DAY ONE: MONDAY

Welcome to day one of the Naturally Thin Program. You can start this program on any day you choose, but for the sake of structure, I'm calling it Monday. Think of today as the day you quit dieting and start living—the day you take back the reins and consciously begin eating to be naturally thin.

To help you do this in the best way possible, today I want you to start thinking about rule 1, and really focus on that concept. Although ideally you will eventually incorporate all ten rules into your daily life, you know as well as I do that drastic changes don't usually work. So, in the spirit of taking baby steps toward your goal, today let's focus on just this: *your diet is a bank account.* It's rule 1, and truthfully, it's the most important habit to change and to make a part of your everyday life and your dietary consciousness.

Your diet is a bank account.

Balancing the foods you eat is really mostly a matter of getting accustomed to doing it. It's not hard or complicated, but you'll have to do it *on purpose* at first. Eventually, it will become second nature. So, without obsessing, I want you mentally to take note of what you eat, why you eat it, and how you feel during and after a meal. Ask yourself what kind of investment you made, how you felt about it, where it fits into your portfolio. Was it a carb meal? A protein meal? A sweet? Was it a good choice? You don't have to write any of this down if you don't want to write it down. In my experience, "keeping a food diary" doesn't work for most people, because most people don't have the time or the inclination to do it. I say, just keep the information in your head. However, if you prefer writing down what you eat and how you feel when you eat it, then I'm not going to argue. It's your life, your body, your food choices, so do what works for *you*.

No matter which way you go about it, I want you to notice everything about your dietary habits today. What do you really want to eat? Do you usually choose to eat what you want, or do you tell yourself you can't have what you want and then have something else instead? What things do you eat that feel more like habit than desire?

But that's not all. Not only do I want you to think about what you've had for one meal; I also want you to think about how each choice you make will work to balance what you will have at the next meal. Don't stress out or obsess about meals to come. Focus more on what you will eat when it's time to eat, and what you really *want* to eat. But when the next meal or snack comes along, remember what you ate before. How will your choices now be influenced by your choices at the last meal? Today you will balance your checkbook and put your eating finances in good working order. You're not dieting anymore. You are living your life. It's easier than you think. Let's start with breakfast.

HEAVY HABIT

Are you in the habit of thinking, "I ate sugar! That was bad! Oh, well, I guess I might as well eat more"? This is destructive thinking, full of self-loathing. You don't deserve this kind of treatment. First of all, if you really want something sweet, you should have it. Have just a little; don't go overboard. Eating too much of any one thing is bad for your body and hard on your digestion, and sugary foods have so many calories that you shouldn't be loading up on them.

Second, if you did mess up and eat too much, why use that as an excuse to eat more? That's just wrong, backward thinking. If anything, eating too much sugar is an excuse to be kinder to yourself by eating more lightly and choosing healthier foods. Be nice! Stop beating yourself up. Do what is ♡ *good for you*. ♡ Acknowledge what you did, add it to your budget, and balance your account by making up for the excess at the next opportunity. Meanwhile, calm down. You're fine.

Day One Breakfast

What do you like to eat for breakfast? Are you a person who craves salty eggs and bacon, and toast with butter? Do you like a huge bakery bagel with cream cheese? Or maybe you are like me and love muffins and other breakfast sweets. Some people like cold cereal, or live for a bowl of hot oatmeal. Or maybe you don't like to eat in the morning but the world has forced you into eating breakfast because it's "the most important meal of the day." You might always want the same thing for breakfast, or your food mood might change each day. But today, I want you to figure out what you really *want* to eat. Right here, right now. Listen to your food voice and remember that no food is forbidden. Breakfast sets your pace for the day.

Maybe you've decided you want something sweet, or you are going

NATURALLY THIN THOUGHT

You might be surprised how hard it is to figure out what you really want, if you aren't used to thinking that way. It's time to start listening to your own body and your own desires. Listen to your food voice. And remember: *You can have it all, just not all at once.*

This can be tricky. You might have to sit quietly for a few minutes and really pay attention to how you feel. What really, truly sounds good to eat? If you aren't sure what you want, wait until you know before you eat. There's no rush, and there is nothing wrong with sitting with your hunger for a while until your food voice defines it more clearly for you, as in: "I thought I should eat wheat toast but I really want a pancake" or "I thought I should eat an egg-white omelet but I really want a fried egg with bacon."

Or you might realize you don't want anything. I used to eat breakfast every morning, the minute I got out of bed, because I just assumed I must be hungry. Breakfast—it's what you do, right? Especially if you are dieting. Studies show that people who eat breakfast lose more weight, blah blah blah. Well, I have a study for you: study yourself. I did, and I realized that eating breakfast when I wasn't hungry was a heavy habit and made me feel hungry all day long. Sometimes I am hungry, and I enjoy the breakfast I really want. But if I'm not hungry, I wait until I am slightly hungry but not so starving that I lose control. It's the only way to get in touch with your food voice and figure out what you really want. If you wake up and you don't want food, don't eat food until you do want it. But if you do want food, eat food. *Know thyself.*

to skip breakfast today, or you're eyeing some leftovers. But for the bacon-and-egg people, today I'm going to talk about savory breakfasts. If you want more guidance right now for some other kind of breakfast, look ahead: if you want something sweet, look at the section about breakfast on day two, Tuesday. If you are a cereal person, look ahead to Wednesday. If you are a bagel or muffin person, go to Thursday. If you like nontraditional breakfasts (such as leftovers from dinner), or if you don't like to eat breakfast at all, check out Friday.

But now, let's talk about bacon and eggs.

For Savory-Breakfast People

If you are a bacon-and-eggs type of breakfast person, think about how you can get what you want and still make the naturally thin choice. Do you want two scrambled eggs with a slice of whole-grain toast? That sounds good. If you eat this, you've deposited plenty of protein in your account, so you really don't need the bacon. But if you are craving bacon, have just one scrambled egg and one slice of turkey bacon with your toast.

I'm talking about balance here. You want to balance all the aspects of your meal so you don't take in too much of any one thing. This includes fat. If you want butter on your toast and you make your eggs at home, use nonstick cooking spray to cook the eggs. Butter is delicious, but you don't need to put it on everything. If you order the eggs in a restaurant, you can bet they'll probably be cooked in butter or oil, so in this case, skip the butter on your toast and use an all-fruit spread instead. Balance. Not sacrifice.

Also remember the concept of the *differential*. You can tweak your breakfast to make it even healthier by omitting things that don't really matter to you, giving yourself more leeway for other, more decadent choices that do matter. For example:

- Some people need and want the whole egg. Others are fine with egg whites. If you like egg whites, go ahead and have two or three. Egg whites have a lot of protein, have virtually no fat, and fill you up, so they are a good investment. If you want the yolks, have less.
- Another option, if you like it, is turkey or veggie bacon or sausage. This is what I usually choose, because to me the *differen-*

167

tial is negligible. The difference in taste between turkey bacon and regular bacon isn't worth the difference in calories and fat. To *me*, turkey bacon is crunchy and salty and just fine. Maybe to you, only real bacon or sausage will do, and that's fine, too, as long as you realize you should only eat a small amount. One slice of bacon and one egg are plenty of protein and fat. If you like the taste, soy or tempeh bacon has even less fat and lots of flavor. But remember, eat what you really *want*, not what you think you are supposed to eat or even what I eat. These choices are up to you. Listen to your food voice.

- Another great way to tweak your eggs is to add lots of filling, high-volume, fiber-rich, nutrient-dense vegetables. Mix them into scrambled eggs or fold them into an omelet. Salsa counts, too. Vegetables fill you up with very few calories, and they can add a lot of extra flavor and interest to your breakfast, which will satisfy you and make you less likely to be hungry again in an hour. They help you balance your account so you can have the foods you want and still be naturally thin.

BETHENNY BYTES

I often wake up thirsty and want just fruit or some juice, but this morning I wanted protein. That's just the kind of day it was. I didn't get a chance to have breakfast until 10:30, and then I had ⅔ of a well-done spinach, mushroom, feta, and egg-white omelette. It was the perfect combo. The only fat was the feta and whatever fat was necessary to cook the eggs. I had this in a restaurant, which probably used butter or oil. If you make this at home, you could certainly use cooking spray. This very satisfying and filling breakfast (even though I left ⅓ of it because what I ate was enough) will allow me to have something sweet later, and you know I will!

Day One Snack

If you aren't a snacker and you aren't hungry between meals, forget the snacks. They certainly aren't required. But if you decide that you will do better with snacks, that's fine. I appreciate the medical findings that support eating five or six small meals every day to keep your blood sugar even and your metabolism stoked. However, I find it anxiety-producing to have to look at my watch to make sure I'm eating every four hours.

I don't snack by the clock, and I recommend that you snack because your food voice says you need a snack, not because it's some specific hour like 10 a.m. or time for your coffee break at work. If you are one of those people who will eat everything in sight because hunger sneaks up on them, then you are a person who needs to snack. *Know thyself,* but also remember that every day will be different. You might need a snack one day, and not the next. *Snacking should not be a habit.*

On days when I snack, I usually try to have a sweet for one of my snacks and a savory for the other. For example, at mid-morning I might have a small whole-grain cookie. If I know I won't make it to dinner, I'll grab a handful of nuts in the afternoon, but really just a small handful. Nuts have a lot of fat, but the fat and protein keep you full for a long time, and that's a good investment. Have a few nuts, give it a beat, have some water, and notice how long this snack stays with you. Don't go hungry, and you won't go crazy later. Nuts are one of the best snacks for me because they help me get through to the next meal, staying in control.

If you are hungry between meals today, after breakfast and before lunch, base your snack on what you had for breakfast, but in general I believe a snack should *always contain some protein.* A piece of fruit isn't going to mitigate your hunger. Have nuts, whole-grain bread with nut butter, a piece of cheese, or some yogurt with your fruit, if that's what you want.

BETHENNY BYTES

After my filling, protein-rich breakfast, sure enough, I was craving something sweet later in the day. I knew I wouldn't have a chance to eat lunch until late, so at about 1 p.m., I had a small bowl of low-fat Ben & Jerry's fudge brownie ice cream. Perfect! I had a very small serving, in a ramekin-sized bowl, and didn't finish it all, and that was just right—not so much that I would have a sugar crash or feel too full and tired, but just enough to make me feel that I had a treat. By the way, I choose low-fat ice cream because for me, the *differential* between a good, all-natural low-fat ice cream like Ben & Jerry's and regular ice cream is nothing. Not all low-fat ice cream is worth it, though. Read the label and avoid the ones full of artificial ingredients. A small scoop of the real stuff is better than a big bowl of the fake stuff any day.

Day One Lunch

For lunch, again, think about what you *really want*, but also think about what you've had for breakfast and whether you had a snack. If you had eggs with turkey bacon, for example, and you *haven't had bread yet,* you might want something like:

- Half a sandwich with soup or salad
- Small serving of pasta loaded with high fiber vegetables
- 1 crab cake (appetizer portion; add a salad)
- Veggie burger (add a salad)
- Small quesadilla with tons of vegetables, preferably on a whole-grain, tomato, or spinach tortilla
- 1 slice of pizza with vegetables

However, if you had carbs for breakfast already—say, a whole wheat pancake, muffin, or toast for breakfast—then you've already had carbs and you need some protein. Think about a protein-dense meal:

- Chicken salad with greens
- Vegetarian chili with a small salad
- Grilled salmon with greens
- Tuna salad with whole-grain crackers and vegetable soup
- Turkey burger with greens, no bun
- Grilled tofu with greens

Notice how I keep suggesting salad or greens. Greens are a super-nutrient-dense, fiber-rich way to fill up, so add them whenever you can. But to go with your greens, choose the food that sounds really good to you, and make sure it will satisfy you. No matter what you eat, if you really wanted something else, it's not going to do the trick.

So what do you want for lunch? What is your food voice telling you? Were you impulsive, indulgent, nutritionally unbalanced at breakfast? Your food noise might be saying, *I was bad at breakfast; I ate sugar; I might as well give up and have more.* But your food voice knows you aren't bad. It's probably telling you how you need to take care of yourself by balancing that sweet breakfast with protein, so listen. *Pay attention!*

If you ate a solid, good-investment breakfast, maybe you want to indulge yourself a little more at lunch—say, with pasta or half a cheeseburger on whole-grain bread (do you need to eat the whole cheeseburger?). Or maybe you're having one of those days where you are going to choose low-calorie, high-fiber choices all day and you don't need any indulgence. Or you don't need it yet. Listen. Can I emphasize this enough? Your food voice is talking. It's telling you what you want.

I often eat lunch out, and when I do, I usually want to eat lightly because I'm in the middle of a busy day and I want to keep my energy up. That's when I turn to the appetizer portion of the lunch menu. So let's talk about appetizers today. You may not be hungry today at lunchtime, and that's fine. Wait until you are hungry and have a snack or some soup. This is not cookie-cutter advice, and only you know what you want. But let's say you do want to order an appetizer.

Whether you are eating out or cooking at home, you can choose appetizer-type foods for lunch, like these:

- Non-creamy soup such as tomato, vegetable, or chicken noodle
- Salad with chicken, feta cheese, and nuts (I always skip the croutons—they seem like a big waste of calories and carbs to me, because I don't really enjoy them)
- Any of the appetizer-type foods I've already mentioned, like a crab cake (one of my favorites), a small quesadilla, stuffed mushrooms, tiny taquitos, or a small portion of fried calamari (another one of my favorites that I used to forbid myself but now enjoy in small portions) along with a salad. Eat whatever sounds good to you and *balances with your breakfast.*

Remember to be a little careful with appetizers, though. Avoid huge appetizers that are deep-fat-fried or drowning in cheese. You know those aren't a good investment. If you think you really want something like that, first fill up on something healthy like a salad or soup. Then and only then, taste the fattening appetizer. These

---

NATURALLY THIN THOUGHT

Sometimes, no matter what you had for breakfast, you are going to really want something that doesn't necessarily balance. Say you had a bagel for breakfast, and now you are craving a slice of pizza or some pasta. That's OK. It happens to everyone. Have half the pasta or one slice of the pizza, but make sure you add a salad or a green vegetable for fiber, volume, and nutrition. Just don't eat all of that fattening food you are craving. Participate in the meal but reduce your portion size. Remember rule 5: ♡ *Downsize now!* ♡ That way, you won't feel deprived, and you'll have the energy and contentment to balance your dinner choices with the first part of your day.

choices aren't off-limits, but you have to be realistic. Participate in the food—taste it, but don't fill up on it, and remember to balance. If one appetizer is fried, or has cheese, or is wrapped in bacon, your other choices should consist of different foods, like vegetables and lean protein.

If the big plate of nachos or pizza or whatever it is you ordered turns out to be too tempting after your taste, give it to someone else at your table or ask the server to pack it up.

Also remember that once you make your decision, you can offer bites of your food to anyone you might be sitting with, and always leave at least two bites of anything you are eating. Remember, you have ♡ *canceled your membership in the Clean Plate Club.* ♡ This is very important! You are cultivating a new way of managing your meals, and losing the heavy habit that tells you to finish every last bit of your food. Listen to your food voice and stop eating when you've had enough and the food doesn't taste exciting anymore. It's the new you, and all those two-bite piles of food *not* going into your mouth are going to add up fast—you'll see. It's like money in the bank.

BETHENNY BYTES

I run around like a lunatic most of the time, and today I didn't get a chance to eat lunch until about 4 p.m. Being really busy actually helps keep me thin. People tend to think that being busy means they have to survive on junk food, but that's just not true. If you eat well when you do eat, then being a busy person can work for you instead of against you.

So what did I eat? I stopped into a Japanese restaurant and had a big bowl of soup loaded with vegetables, chicken, and soba noodles. However, I didn't eat all the noodles; I mostly ate just the vegetables, chicken, and broth. I also had some edamame and a salad. I felt energized and satisfied afterward. If I had eaten all those noodles, I would have filled up on a worse investment. Better to fill up on broth and eat fewer noodles. Just because you have noodles in your bowl doesn't mean you have to eat every single one!

Day One Dinner

When it's time for a dinner, a lot of people have the mentality that it's time to eat a lot of food. That's just a heavy habit. You don't have to eat a lot of food to eat good food that you really want. Less is more.

How you handle dinner will depend, to some extent, on where you eat. Are you going out to a restaurant, or are you eating at home? See Friday (day five) for more on how to eat the naturally thin way in a restaurant. Today, let's talk about eating at home.

Ironically, I think it's sometimes easier to maintain control at a restaurant because when you look at a menu, you have a premeditated choice and you also have controlled portions. You order something wise and you bring home leftovers, getting two meals for the price of one.

But at home, especially if you are eating with children, controlling your portions can be more challenging. You've got a refrigerator and a pantry full of food. So we have to plan this out methodically.

First of all, let's set a few ground rules for cooking at home.

1. Don't Snack While Cooking!

You can eat an entire meal's worth of food just by nibbling while you cook. Then you sit down to another meal. That's a heavy habit to break right now. You need to taste the food you are cooking to make sure it's good and to adjust seasonings. That's OK, and a lot different from eating chips and guacamole the whole time you are making enchiladas.

In other words, grazing while cooking is a no-no. Do you need somebody to forbid you to do this? Fine. I hereby *forbid you to graze while cooking.* You do not need those sneaky, unsatisfying calories that don't feel as if you ate anything, right before you are about to sit down to a nice meal. Instead, sip a glass of water while you cook.

2. Always Start with a Salad

Throughout the week, I'll talk about various components of dinner. Go to Tuesday (day two) for more about bread with dinner; go to Wednesday (day three) for my thoughts on pasta (I have a lot of thoughts on pasta); and check out Thursday (day four) for more about protein-based entrées. But today, let's begin at the beginning of this meal and talk about salad.

NATURALLY THIN THOUGHT

A lot of diet books tell you to get your salad dressing "on the side." I don't agree. When I see people do this, I notice that they usually end up dipping everything in the dressing and eating it all. Instead, just dress your salad *lightly,* or ask the restaurant to do it for you. You don't want greens dripping in dressing, but a freshly prepared, lightly dressed salad is fantastic, and you'll probably end up eating less dressing than you would have been given on the side. Do I have to tell you that vinaigrette is a better investment than creamy dressing? A little olive oil, lemon juice, salt, and pepper make an excellent, simple, pure, dressing.

I consider a salad not only a delicious way to eat vegetables full of fiber and nutrients, but a tool for being naturally thin. Every night, before you eat one single thing for dinner, have a salad.

If you get tired of salad, get more creative. Salads don't have to be boring, and they certainly don't have to be the same every day. Shake things up. Here are some ideas:

- Choose dark leafy greens like arugula, spinach, and mesclun for your salad. These greens have more flavor and need less dressing than plain iceberg lettuce, which is mostly water and not very nutritious. Romaine is better, but still not as nutrient-dense or flavorful as some of the other greens. Remember: the darker the color, the better.

- Add colorful, exciting vegetables to your salad. I like to make salads completely from leftover herbs, such as parsley, basil, cilantro, dill, and a few bitter greens like watercress and arugula. Add pear tomatoes for color. Chop orange and red peppers for tangy crunch. Use a carrot peeler and put some carrot shavings on top. Get excited about your salad, as if it were a work of art.
- I also like to choose one or two fun ingredients for my salad. Maybe it's a certain toasted nut, like pecans or pine nuts, combined with a lower-fat, higher-flavor cheese like Parmesan, feta, or blue cheese. To me, that makes a salad even more interesting. By the way, you don't need very much of these high-flavor cheeses to add a lot of character to your salad.
- Finally, don't let yourself get stuck in a salad rut. You might love a certain mix of greens, veggies, and nuts, but vary it for better nutrition and excitement. One night, try arugula, sun-dried tomatoes, and goat cheese with olive oil and lemon. Another day, try baby spinach, walnuts, and tomatoes with raspberry vinaigrette. You can mix in some Asian greens (sold in bags and at some farmers markets) and sprinkle sesame seeds on top. Make your own Asian vinaigrette of olive oil, a dash of sesame oil, honey, lime, and soy sauce.

The point is to have the salad, eat it before you eat anything else, fill up on that first, and include your family. They should all be eating salads, too, right? It's better for digestion, not to mention discipline, if everyone sits down together and calmly enjoys a salad at the beginning of every meal, before moving on to the next part of the meal. Make salad a habit.

You can always tweak your salad choices to make them even better, if the *differential* is negligible. Some ideas:

- Keep downsizing the amount of oil in your vinaigrette. Use the least amount that still satisfies your taste, but don't use so little that you don't like the result. Find your perfect oil-to-vinegar ratio. No fake dressing. No lemon-salt-pepper is your new best friend.

- As often as you can, include a new kind of vegetable or leafy green in your salad. You'll expand your nutrient profile while also expanding your palate and food knowledge. You'll be able to offer an informed opinion about mizuna or escarole, or whether you prefer watercress, arugula, or dandelion greens.

BETHENNY BYTES

Tonight I had dinner at 8 p.m. By then, I was quite hungry. I ordered a large garden salad with cucumbers, tomatoes, and tons of other veggies. I also had a little bit of crumbled feta and some lightly marinated Italian vegetables on top. I ate the whole salad first to fill up.

Next, I had half a turkey burger. I ate only half because it wasn't very good (I ordered this at a diner). There is no reason to waste calories on food that doesn't thrill you. It's not worth. I'd rather spend those calories elsewhere. I had no bun, because I chose to have half a baked potato instead, and I skipped the cheese on the burger because I had chosen to have feta on my salad. See how that keeps me in balance? The turkey burger and the feta contained protein to keep me satisfied, and all those veggies really filled me up. Aside from the inferior turkey burger (I would have preferred something that tasted better), this dinner was a good investment. This was also one of those meals evenly split between protein and carbs, so I consider it a carb/protein combo meal.

Day One Late-Night Snacking

Sometimes, you will be hungry later in the evening, after dinner. Sometimes you won't be. It's important not to eat an evening snack just because you always eat one. That's a waste. Listen to your food voice. If you really want something, have it. Just don't have very much. If you know nighttime eating sets you off and you won't be able to stop, then don't start. ♡ *Know thyself.* ♡ Hold off for a few weeks until you break this heavy habit. But remember to tell yourself that you can snack at night again soon, after you've retrained the part that makes you lose control. You are in charge of what you eat!

I often crave something sweet in the evening, although not always. When I do, I have what I want, such as low-fat ice cream. Ice cream isn't a bad choice when you are craving sweets, because it has protein and calcium. I choose low-fat ice cream, but only the kinds made from real ingredients, not a bunch of artificial fillers. Read the label. Low-fat is a good choice because you might have a hard time digesting a lot of fat late at night. Ben & Jerry's is one of my favorites because it has a list of ingredients I understand.

If you like sorbet or granita (not sherbet, which is often full of fat), that's even better. Sorbet and granita are like ice cream but are made with fruit, ice, and sugar. They have no fat and far fewer calories than ice cream and frozen yogurt, but they have intense flavor. They are vegan (containing no animal products, including dairy), in case that matters to you.

No matter which sweet snack you choose, have just a little cup. Remember the small ramekins in Chapter 5? That's the size of the bowl you want for your late-night snacking.

Maybe you crave salty snacks like popcorn or one of those soft pretzels with cheese sauce, or you just want a little more of what you had for dinner. That's fine, too. Your food voice will tell you what you want. Just have a little, to be kind to your body. You'll sleep better.

You did it—you got through the first day of the Naturally Thin Program. You've left dieting behind for good and you've started living as a naturally thin person. How do you feel? If you are used to stuffing yourself or depriving yourself, you probably feel both light and satisfied. That's the feeling you will have most of the time when you follow the Naturally Thin Program. And it feels great.

BETHENNY BYTES

At about 10 this evening, I wanted something sweet, so I had a small bowl of low-fat granola with soymilk and dried blueberries. It's what I really wanted, so it was perfect.

Or maybe you're struggling a little, just because you are so *used* to eating in an imbalanced way. That's fine, too. Heavy habits take a while to break, but you are getting there. You are driving now, remember? You are the one in charge of your own life. If you didn't eat exactly the way you intended today, it's OK. This is a process.

Sometimes you'll have PMS or feel bloated or be starving or stressed out because of what's going on in your life. Sometimes you'll be more tempted to overindulge. At other times, you won't be hungry at all. This is life, and when you eat to be naturally thin, you do it while living your life, so we're not going to pretend those things don't happen. This was just one day, and there will be many, many others, with thousands of opportunities for making choices about what you want to eat and what you choose not to eat. You're already learning to choose well. Good job!

Day One Recipes

A simple frittata for breakfast is an easy and elegant way to enjoy eggs. For lunch, try my all-time fave sandwich—tofu salad. For dinner, make a traditional Caesar salad that's even better than the versions in restaurants because it's fresher and lower in fat.

Idiot-Proof Delicious Tofu Salad Sandwich

This is one of my absolute favorite things to eat, and so quick to make, too.

7 ounces firm tofu, drained and mashed with a fork (I like Nasoya brand—it comes
  water-packed in a plastic box)

1 teaspoon Dijon mustard

1 teaspoon mayonnaise (if you prefer, choose low-fat or soy mayonnaise)

¾ teaspoon Spike seasoning (You can replace this with salt and pepper, but at some
  point you have to try Spike. It is life-changing.)

Combine all the ingredients and spread on a toasted scooped bagel or
a slice of toasted Ezekial sprouted grain bread with a slice of soy cheese
or veggie cheese. I usually finish the whole thing. Tofu is high in protein and it's not going to make you fat.

Easy Impressive Frittata

This fancy-looking but super-easy recipe makes a beautiful and healthful
breakfast.

Serves 1 (Double the recipe and use a medium-size pan to serve 2.)

Cooking spray

1 cup sautéed vegetables (great way to use leftovers), such as onions, spinach,
  zucchini, broccoli, or tomatoes

1 egg yolk and 3 to 4 egg whites

Salt and pepper, to taste

1 tablespoon crumbled feta or grated Parmesan

1. Preheat the oven to 350°F. Spray a small nonstick pan with an
ovenproof handle with cooking spray. Over medium heat, sauté the
vegetables.

2. In a small bowl, whisk together the egg yolk and egg whites with
a little salt and pepper. Pour the egg mixture into the pan and move it
around with a spatula until slightly solidified. Transfer the pan to the
oven.

3. Bake until the frittata is almost firm to the touch (approximately

15 to 20 minutes). Sprinkle with the cheese and bake until firm. Serve immediately.

Old School Caesar Salad

This is a delicious and quick Caesar salad.

Serves 2

4 cups chopped romaine, well washed

1 teaspoon Dijon mustard

½ teaspoon minced garlic

2 tablespoons freshly squeezed lemon juice

1 teaspoon anchovy paste

2 teaspoons Worcestershire sauce

4 tablespoons extra-virgin olive oil

3 tablespoons grated Parmesan

Salt and pepper, to taste

1. Put the lettuce in a large bowl. In a jar, combine mustard, garlic, lemon juice, anchovy paste, Worcestershire sauce, and olive oil. Shake until combined.

2. Drizzle the dressing over the lettuce. Sprinkle with Parmesan and season with salt and pepper. Toss well to completely coat the lettuce. Serve immediately.

Chapter 13

DAY TWO: TUESDAY

Today is day two of the Naturally Thin Program, but also just another day in your life. Another Tuesday, and another day of living naturally thin. Remember, you are *not* on a diet anymore, nor will you ever be again. You're just working on some new habits, and this is a day in your (new) normal life.

Today, I would like you to keep thinking about the concept that *your diet is a bank account,* and I also want you to start thinking seriously about rule 2: *pay attention.* Today, be conscious about what, when, how, and why you eat. Taste every bite and don't you dare even think about watching television, sitting at your computer, or talking on the phone while eating. You can't possibly pay attention to your food when you do these things, and you want to make every bite count.

Let's start with breakfast.

Day Two Breakfast

I talked about savory breakfasts yesterday, so today, let's begin by talking directly to the people who like a sweet breakfast. I'm one of you, so believe me, I know what it feels like to wake up and crave something sweet. However, once you get into the habit of including a little protein when you eat sweets, you will feel your cravings decreasing. Protein helps break the sugar habit. It doesn't happen to me every morning and it won't happen to you every morning, but let's talk about what to do when it does happen.

For Sweet-Breakfast People

If you love sweet, carb-laden breakfasts, I can relate to that. This is my favorite kind of breakfast. Maybe you want pancakes, a muffin, or a pastry. That's fine. Here's how to do it.

If you want a pastry, stop and think how it will make you feel afterward. What do you have going on today and how will your choice affect you? Is it going to ruin your day, making you tired and cranky? If so, is it really worth the momentary pleasure? Or, when you think of the big picture, would you rather make a more nutrient-dense choice that really feels as though it's worth the calories? If you can handle it, have half of, say, a doughnut or a chocolate croissant or whatever you like, but add some semblance of protein. Even better, have just two or three bites, but if you are going to do this, *know and understand that it is not a good investment.* You can still eat it if you want it. But you will need to invest more wisely at your next opportunity, balancing this choice with the rest of your choices for the day.

Also realize that if you have something sweet now, it means skipping something sweet later. Which do you want more? Make your choice. *You can have it all, just not all at once.* Are you willing to give up dessert or a cocktail tonight? Or ice cream in the mid-afternoon? Tomorrow you might do things differently, but today, choose and decide which way you want to go. And you can have it both ways, too—remember the concept of two exceptions? If you have just one or two bites of a pastry, you can still have sweets later. It's just a taste. When it comes to really decadent treats, remember to ♡ *taste everything, eat nothing.*♡ Really savor that one bite (or two bites), then throw away or give away the rest.

If you are going to do this—whether you commit yourself to a sweet breakfast or have just a taste—you have to do one other thing: have some protein. Without the protein to slow down the absorption of all that sugar, you'll probably crash later. Protein will help this breakfast stay with you longer, so have some walnuts, yogurt, or cottage cheese, or part skim ricotta. (Also see Chapter 15 for more information on muffin/bagel breakfasts.)

Maybe you decide to forget the doughnut. That doesn't mean you're going to forget your craving for something sweet. If you want a pancake or waffle, by all means have one big one or two small ones. Eating a pancake or waffle in the right way can be a good investment. But you don't need a big stack of them. If you really eat consciously, paying attention to every bite, one or two will be plenty.

Whole-grain pancakes and waffles stick with you longer and give you more fiber and nutrition than those made with white flour, and they taste great, too. Choose your sweet topping sensibly: is it a drizzle of real maple syrup (not the fake high-fructose corn-syrup junk) or agave syrup? Maybe you like a sprinkle of raw sugar, or some all-fruit spread with a few walnuts or sliced almonds, or a dollop of yogurt with fresh berries. Adding fresh fruit to your pancake or waffle will help fill you up because you are getting the whole, juicy, fresh, fiber-rich fruit. Adding fresh fruit and protein like nuts or yogurt will keep you full longer.

Don't do it all, though. Don't add maple syrup, yogurt, nuts, and fruit. ♡ *You can have it all, just not all at once.*♡

Fruity Breakfasts

Maybe fresh juicy fruit sounds just right. Fruit is a great choice for breakfast, especially if you wake up feeling thirsty, or if you overindulged the day before. Fruit has a cleansing, refreshing effect on your body, and it also tastes sweet. So if that sounds good to you, have a bowl of fruit—preferably whatever is in season when possible, because that will taste best and be most nutritious.

Don't forget that although fruit is full of vitamins, it also has a high natural sugar content, so if you don't eat it with protein, you will probably be hungry soon after. Sometimes, I want only fruit for breakfast, but then I usually need a late-morning snack. Eat fruit, but recognize what that might mean for your hunger level. A little bit of protein in the form of yogurt, a few walnuts, or some cheese will really improve a meal of fruit.

BETHENNY BYTES

I woke up feeling dehydrated from the alcohol I had at a party the night before, plus a lack of sleep. OK, I admit I was hungover. What I really wanted when I woke up was sliced watermelon from the deli, so I went out to get some. That's when I saw the hot chocolate machine. In the old days, I would have limited myself to fat-free, fake-sugar-flavored hot chocolate and added more sweetener and felt disgusted. Not now. I bought some watermelon. Then I took the smallest cup the deli had, filled it with the rich, creamy hot chocolate, and decided it was going to be a sugar breakfast.

Was that a nutritionally balanced breakfast? Not even close. I knew I would be hungry later. But that was my day today and that was the breakfast I really wanted today. Everybody has days like this, and this is why it doesn't make sense to try to stick to a preset diet plan. I made an impulsive decision because of something I really wanted, but I did it with a conscious willingness to give up something else later. I also recognized that what I drank the night before influenced how I felt at that moment. Every moment connects to the next moment. I decided the hot chocolate was worth it, and I would invest more wisely at lunch to balance out my breakfast splurge. I ate the watermelon, drank the hot chocolate, and moved on to the next thing.

About Coffee

You're probably not going to listen to me when I tell you this, but if just one person listens, I've made a difference. Caffeine is bad for you. It contributes to cravings for sweets, it's dehydrating, and everything people put in it (cream, sugar, or that horrible fake flavored sugary nondairy creamer) makes it even worse.

But I'm a realist. I know that a lot of you are going to keep drinking coffee. I admit I have some once in a while, too, although I usually have just one cup. I like the ritual of a hot cup of coffee. So drink your coffee, but balance your account:

- Can you drink decaf? What's the *differential* for you? If you like decaf and don't care about the caffeine, this is a preferable option. If not, it's something to consider for the future, but I know you might want your coffee fully charged.
- If you like those fancy Starbucks drinks, get one a day, get the smallest one, and consider it one of your daily sweets. You don't have to finish it, either. Have some until you feel satisfied, then throw the rest away. Thin people do that all the time.
- If you drink lattes, understand that the calories really add up in the milk and sugar. Have just one or two a day. Then you'll have to give up something else. You decide what. If you have one latte, fine. If you like it with skim milk, great. If you really want the whole milk, that's fine, too—just remember that you have to balance by giving up something high in fat later. If you really need two lattes to keep you going, then give up a sweet, a piece of bread, a cocktail, or whatever you think seems equal in value to the latte that day. This is balancing.
- If you are unsure about what constitutes a serving of fat or a sweet, simply be sensible about it. If you like black coffee with just a splash of cream that's no big deal. If you like flavored syrup and a lot of cream, well, yes, that counts. Only you know

whether you should categorize your choice of coffee as an indulgence.

* As for obsessing about skim milk over full-fat milk, don't be absurd. We're talking about a spoonful. One tablespoon of half-and-half has 20 calories and less than 2 grams of fat. That's nothing. If you like the taste of your coffee with skim milk, low-fat milk, or soymilk, great. If you really like a dash of cream, fine. The French do it every day, and look how thin they are. But remember, they savor a tiny cappuccino. They aren't drinking the enormous drinks Americans seem to like so much. ♡*Downsize now!*♡ This is an example of quality vs. quantity. I'd rather have a teaspoon of real cream than half a cup of skim milk. Again, it's the *differential*.

NATURALLY THIN THOUGHT

I'm a fan of Synergy Kombucha, a naturally fermented, raw bottled drink. It helps control my appetite, improves my digestion, and gives me energy. Some people think it tastes like vinegar, and it is an acquired taste. At first, I thought it was disgusting, frankly. But it contains active enzymes and probiotics (like the kind in yogurt), which really give your immune system a boost and make your whole body work better. Now I'm addicted. I have one almost every day for breakfast. Kombucha is expensive, but to me, the benefits are worth the expense. I've reduced my coffee consumption, and only drink decaf, now that I drink Kombucha. It has a tart taste, and is very thirst-quenching. I like the brand Synergy, which contains ninety-five percent Kombucha and five percent fresh juice, like cranberry, raspberry, grape, or ginger.

By the way, when I drink Synergy Kombucha, I don't count it as anything. It has 80 calories, but it's just something I decided to include in my life. Maybe your thing is that extra cup of coffee, iced tea, or whatever. Sometimes, things can be "free." Don't obsess!

Day Two Lunch

I often find it hard to make time for lunch because I'm so busy. But instead of grabbing junk food on the run, I try to make time to eat something that will help me get through the rest of the day productively. One of my favorite quick lunches is soup.

Soup fills you up, the vegetables are nutritious, and the protein stays with you. I usually try to avoid soup with a lot of noodles or rice because the broth, protein, and vegetables are what fill me up and make me feel healthy and strong. I also avoid cream soups because they are very high in fat and the *differential* doesn't seem worth it to me. You might like cream soup, but if you do, have just a little. Once you start listening to your body, you'll feel how quickly a bowl of pureed vegetable soup fills you up, and you won't even miss the cream.

I also like soup because it is comfort food. A lot of people eat for comfort. Why pretend that this doesn't happen? It's human nature. That's one reason I think soup is a wonder food, especially for people with weight issues. Even pureed vegetables are comforting, and they can help get you through the day; you feel that you are nurturing yourself without taking in a lot of calories and fat. One of my favorite soups, especially in the summer, is gazpacho. I think it's just about the world's most perfect food.

In general, look for broth-based soup—in other words, soup that isn't swimming with cream. There should be tons of veggies and some lean protein such as chicken, fish, or tofu. If the soup has just a splash of milk or cream, that's fine—have a small cup. But you know what I mean by cream soup—New England clam chowder, potato cheese, soups like that. Those are definitely soups to taste, not eat. If you are really hungry, you might choose chili. I skip the cheese and sour cream on top, but a dollop of salsa and a few cubes of avocado make a really good topping.

I'm a fan of turkey or veggie chili because it gives me all the spicy chili taste without all the fatty meat. You can make chili at home using ground turkey or veggie crumbles, or just leave those out and use lots of high-fiber beans, such as black beans and pinto beans. Of course, you also want to fill your chili with vegetables, because they will fill *you* up. See my recipe for Ultra-Healthy Mexican Chili at the end of this chapter.

Some people rely on canned or boxed soup for lunch, especially when they are crunched for time. I understand that, and I'm not going to be a hypocrite and say I never eat canned soup, because I do. I also love the boxed soups by Imagine and Pacific Natural Foods. But when I do choose canned or boxed soup, I look at the list of ingredients. I choose organic soups with real ingredients instead of soups with a lot of fillers and things I can't pronounce. When you choose wisely, canned soup can be a quick practical choice.

However, if you do have the time and inclination, nothing beats homemade soup for taste and nutrition. It also contains less sodium, because you control the ingredients. Homemade soup is also a great way to repurpose leftover veggies and meat. You can make a big batch of homemade soup on a weekend, then freeze individual portions to microwave for lunch all week and combine with half a sandwich or a slice of bread and a slice of cheese.

BETHENNY BYTES

Today for lunch, I wanted something savory, so I had a medium-sized bowl of chicken noodle soup with large pieces of white-meat chicken and a small amount of noodles. I ate some of the noodles, but not all of them—just enough to keep me satisfied. I also had half an Idiot-Proof Delicious Tofu Salad Sandwich (see the recipe on page 180).

If you choose soup for lunch but it doesn't seem like enough, think about what you had for breakfast. If you had something high-carb like a pancake or muffin, skip bread with your soup, and add a salad with some protein, especially if you know you'll want something starchy for dinner. If you had eggs or something more protein-based for breakfast and you really want a slice of bread with your soup, go ahead. Whole-grain bread is the best, most nutritious, most filling choice. Or consider having a small salad with your soup. You can't eat too many veggies. You could also have an apple, a pear, or some other kind of fruit you like for dessert, if you didn't already load up on fruit at breakfast. Remember, fruit is good for you, but even healthy foods (except raw vegetables) have to be balanced throughout the day if you want to be naturally thin.

HEAVY HABIT

I often hear people say, "I'm eating a light lunch because I'm going out for a big dinner." This is absurd. You might feel that this is "balancing," but too often the logic backfires. You don't eat enough at lunch, so you are starving and then you eat way too much in one sitting at dinner. If you know what you will be having for dinner, then you can make choices at lunch that will balance those dinner foods. Plan and manage your investments. You are an adult. You don't have to skip lunch. Eat lunch, in order to go to dinner without going off the rails. If you know you will be going to one of those restaurants with huge portions that feeds you like an animal, remember that you are *not* an animal and do not have to eat everything they put in front of you.

Starving yourself before a big event isn't living in the moment or listening to your food voice. Don't live by the clock. Instead, know your body. If you eat by the clock or by some idea you have of what's always happening in the future, that's not listening to your food voice. It sets you up for a binge. Living in the moment and making sensible, balanced choices whenever you feel that you need to eat will create a string of good investments and eating experiences leading to an overall healthy lifestyle and natural thinness.

Day Two Snack

Use smart, satisfying snacks to spoil your appetite so you don't ever overindulge at other times. But snacking can also hurt you if you do it purely out of habit or boredom or just because you happen to be sitting at your desk or watching television. That's a no-no, right? You know now to ♡ *pay attention.*♡

On those days when you do crave a snack, have one. Think about whether you had a morning snack, and if so what kind of snack it was. Remember to balance a savory snack with a sweet snack, so if you've already had sweets today, forget the mini Snickers bar (you can always choose one tomorrow) and think about what might balance your accounts more wisely. It won't be very long before you will *instinctively* know what to have.

BETHENNY BYTES

After my light lunch of soup, I felt hungry later in the afternoon. Remembering that rich hot chocolate and fruit for breakfast, I knew I wanted to balance this snack with something that wasn't sweet and add protein. Besides, I craved something salty. I was on the go and didn't have much time, so I had a bag of Glenny's Multigrain Soy Crisps. These have simple ingredients, few calories, and 6 grams of protein, which is a lot more than you'll find in most "chips," so they really kept me going until dinner.

Day Two Dinner

Now it's time for dinner, so it's time to consider what you've eaten so far today. That will help guide your choices for this meal. You've got plenty of choices, and I want you to eat what sounds great. But I also want you to think about how your choices will affect you. So today, let's talk about bread.

Bread, to many people, is a staple and they don't think they can live without it. It appears like magic on your table at a restaurant. It comes automatically with all kinds of things you might order, such as scrambled eggs, soup, or roast chicken. People cooking at home might also feel compelled to put some bread on the table, whether it's a baguette, biscuits, dinner rolls, or crackers. Enough, already! Why do people serve garlic bread with spaghetti? It's overkill.

BETHENNY BYTES

Recently, I was out with friends and we didn't get a chance to eat until 10 p.m. I had a SkinnyGirl Margarita, then thought about what I wanted for dinner.

I started with a green salad with vinaigrette. I always make it interesting with extra veggies like tomatoes, pea shoots, or whatever is available. For the appetizer, I ordered a small cheese plate with olives and marinated vegetables. This came with bread, but I skipped the bread because I'd had noodles at lunch and soy crisps for a snack. I also had a drink (counts as a sweet), so I wanted this to be a protein meal. I had a few good, flavorful bites of a friend's buttery New York strip steak and filled up on a combination of two side dishes: sautéed mushrooms and broccoli rabe which was oily but delicious. It was a satisfying and filling dinner because I had filled up on high-volume, high-fiber foods. As a result, I didn't need as much of the decadent foods, but I didn't deprive myself of them, either. Remember: don't deprive yourself by eating only vegetables. It's about balance. I needed those bites of steak, but I didn't need very many of them, and the fact that the steak was on someone else's plate, not mine, helped me listen more rationally to my food voice, which told me I didn't need more than a few bites.

I also have to say here that I realize you won't always be in a situation where somebody else can order an entrée for you to taste. That's fine. This is just how it works for me on occasion. Order what you want, and if you need a smaller portion, ask for one or ask to have part of the meal packed up for you to take home before you even start eating, if that helps you stick to your plan.

I'm not saying bread isn't a good food. A hearty whole-grain bread is nutritious and satisfying. But it's all about balance. If you've been eating carbs all day, you don't need bread for dinner; and if you feel you want it, really think about whether that's just a habit or whether you are actually hungry for it. Is it really *bread* you want, or is it something else, even if you don't know what?

When I'm really in the mood for bread with dinner and I know I haven't had many carbs that day, I'll have some bread, but usually just a small piece of the end with a tiny smear of butter or olive oil or a bit of cheese from my salad. I participated, I stopped, and I don't feel deprived.

Now, you too are a person who is thin and eats whatever she wants. But that doesn't mean that you aren't considering, in the

---

NATURALLY THIN THOUGHT

A few weeks ago, I went to sleep at 2 a.m. because I had been out at a friend's birthday party. I assumed there would be dinner, but there were only fattening hors d'oeuvres, so I opted for two cheese-and-vegetable quesadilla triangles. It looked good, and I knew I would get protein in the cheese and nutrients in the vegetables which was better than the fried shrimp. This would help balance the alcohol in the two SkinnyGirl Margaritas I had (see Chapter 16 for the recipe).

But that's all I had for dinner. It wasn't much of a dinner, but I had a stressful week and hadn't had much of an appetite, and I don't believe in eating just to eat. I'm not telling you to skip meals, because sometimes this can be *very bad for you.* I have gotten to the point where my body tells me when it needs something, and that's a great feeling. Have you heard the old saying, "Feed a cold, starve a fever"? Or maybe it's the other way around. Either way, I don't buy it. Sometimes your body needs to conserve energy for healing, so listen to your food voice, and never force yourself to eat when you are sick, stressed, or just not hungry.

back of your head, your bread allowance for the day. If you already had a turkey sandwich for lunch, you decided then to spend your bread allowance there. Remember that what happened all day affects this meal right now. You made the decisions. And if you simply must have bread anyway, have a small slice lightly dipped in olive oil as one of your daily "exceptions." It will make you feel as though you participated in the entire bread experience, even though you have only a bite or two. You'll feel like everyone else at the table, instead of being the person who is terrified of bread. Nothing is fattening in small quantities.

I remember sitting in a restaurant once, and hearing a crazy woman at a table next to me practically scream at the waiter, "Take this bread off the table!" You don't want to be that person, do you? Relax. Don't fear the bread. It's *bread*. You can participate in the bread if you want to participate in the bread, and still be naturally thin.

Day Two Snack — or Dessert

As long as we're talking about carb-laden foods, let's also talk about dessert. Sometimes, I have a snack at night, and it's often really just a dessert delayed from dinner. I don't like to mix a lot of foods at the same time, so I think that if you are going to have dessert, it's good to wait a little while, if possible, to digest your dinner first.

But either way, you probably know, or think you know, that fruit is a better dessert than a big piece of cake or a bowl of ice cream. This is true—in a way. But let's really look at the whole concept of "fruit for dessert."

When I eat fruit right after a meal, I often feel bloated and uncomfortable. Not everybody agrees with me about this, but I tend to subscribe to the theory that fruit (along with a few nuts) is best eaten on an empty stomach. Your body digests it quickly that way. You feel light and clean when you eat fruit alone, even though it will tend to make you hungry again soon afterward. Fruit is cleansing.

But if you wait a while after dinner, fruit might be just what you want. If you really *want* a bowl of strawberries instead of a bowl of ice cream, absolutely make that choice. But is that really what you want? Are you sure? I'm not saying it isn't, I'm just saying: don't have fruit because you think you are supposed to have fruit, when you really want something else. That is ignoring your food voice. A bowl of fruit is about the same number of calories as a few bites of a rich dessert, so have the one you really want. You have to figure out what the *differential* is. If a bowl of strawberries is just about as good to you as a bowl of strawberry ice cream, go for the strawberries. But if it's not worth it, you'll just feel deprived, and you'll eat more later. Trust me.

Nighttime is a dangerous time for some people to eat. It's a common time to binge, especially if you've deprived yourself all day of the foods you really want. You night eaters know who you are, so please remember: *Check yourself before you wreck yourself.* This is why it's so important to eat the foods you want before the sun goes down and you're suddenly on the rampage, ready to eat everything in sight. If you can easily eat a whole day's worth of calories between 9 p.m. and midnight, you aren't eating to be naturally thin.

You've done it—day two. How do you feel? At the end of this day, think about how your body is doing, and also how your brain is do-

---

BETHENNY BYTES

Tonight, I had to attend an evening party. As usual, there was a large spread, but I looked over everything first to decide what I really wanted. Just as you don't go into a store and buy the first thing you see, you have to shop around in situations like this. Look at everything before you decide what to take to the register (or put in your mouth). Don't let the menu or the buffet drive your choices. You drive. I had already eaten dinner, so I chose a few deviled eggs because they are high in protein, and I had a few sips of delicious champagne. After that, I drank water, to stay hydrated. I knew this would help me feel and look good tomorrow.

ing. Do you feel that you ate enough for your needs? Do you feel fulfilled, or deprived? If you don't feel good or you do feel deprived, you need to eat a little more. It takes some practice, getting used to listening to your food voice, and when you are trying to lose some weight, it's easy to err on the side of undereating because you are still dealing with fear of food. That's perfectly natural. Just keep reminding yourself that *you are not on a diet*.

You need to eat, and you need to eat the foods your body tells you it needs. Your food voice might be telling you not to eat something really good because you don't quite believe me when I say that you can do this and still be OK. But you have to trust me here. You *can* do this. Thin people do it every day. Vow to eat the foods you really want, and to focus on balancing your choices throughout the day. Stay with me. By the end of the week, you'll be hearing your food voice much more clearly. This is a marathon, not a sprint. It took a while to get to this point in your life, and now it will take a while to get where you are going. You aren't going to reach your ideal weight in one day, but you are most definitely on your way.

Day 2 Recipes

Try these easy recipes for fruit skewers and a favorite chili to keep you focused on high flavor and volume without a lot of fat and calories.

Rainbow Fruit Skewers

This beautiful and simple recipe serves as many as you want it to serve. Make two small skewers or one large skewer for each person you are serving.

Line a white platter with fresh blueberries, then put chunks of fruit on wooden skewers in the colors of the rainbow:

Red: Watermelon
Orange: Mango
Yellow: Pineapple

Green: Kiwi

Blue: Blueberries

Purple: Purple grapes

Ultra-Healthy Mexican Chili

This is a popular recipe on my Web site. It substitutes ground turkey for the typical ground beef; or you can just skip the turkey if you want a vegetarian version. If beans bug you, you can even leave those out. It will still be good. This chili also tastes great the next day.

Serves 1 (Double, triple, or quadruple it to serve more people.)

½ medium onion, chopped

Nonstick cooking spray

1 teaspoon chili powder

1 teaspoon cumin

Salt and pepper, to taste

2 cloves garlic, minced

¼ each chopped red and yellow bell pepper (or just chop half a bell pepper of any color)

1 small can (about 8 ounces) of pureed tomatoes or tomato sauce

½ cup zucchini, chopped

¼ pound ground turkey breast

¼ cup canned red pinto beans, drained and rinsed

1. Over medium-high heat, sauté the onion in a nonstick skillet coated in cooking spray until soft. Add the chili powder, cumin, salt, and pepper.

2. Stir in the garlic and bell peppers, and cook until the peppers are soft and the garlic is golden but not burned. Stir in the tomato sauce and the zucchini.

3. When all the vegetables are soft, add the turkey breast and beans. Let the chili simmer for at least 10 or 15 minutes. The longer you simmer, the better the flavor. Serve.

Chapter 14

DAY THREE: WEDNESDAY

On day three of the Naturally Thin Program, you will still be considering your investments, balancing your accounts, and eating consciously. Today I also want you to devote some time to thinking about rule 3: *You can have it all, just not all at once.*

Whenever you make a choice about something you really want to eat, stop there. Pick a lane. Don't focus on what you want *with* what you chose, or what you *don't get* to eat because of your choice. Don't have buyer's remorse. Just go with your choice and enjoy it. You don't need to eat fries and a milkshake with that cheeseburger. You don't need bread and dessert with your pasta. Pick the one best thing, then really enjoy it. You didn't choose something else, because you didn't want something else as much as you wanted what you did choose. Maybe next time you will want something else more, and then you can have that. It's like shopping. You can't have everything, so pick what you want and go with that.

You get it. Nothing is off-limits, so calm down and just enjoy what you've committed to eating *right now*. It's just like in life. We have to choose to focus on what we really want. You don't get George Clooney, Brad Pitt, *and* Justin Timberlake. OK, maybe you don't actually get any of them, but if you did, what would you do with them all? (Don't answer that.) The point is that you pick one gorgeous indulgence. Leave the rest for another time. *You can have it all, just not all at once.*

HEAVY HABIT

Do you ever find yourself thinking, or even saying out loud, "I can't stop eating this!" I remember thinking this all the time. But when I look back, now that I eat to be naturally thin, it couldn't seem more absurd. What do you mean you can't stop eating?

Look, I understand about binging, and I talk about that in Chapter 7. But right now I'm talking about something so many of us do: "Oh, cheesecake! I can't stop." "I just have to eat that prime rib. I don't want to but I just can't help it!" "Hey, what could I do? They were M&Ms."

It's the "you can't have just one" mentality from the potato chip commercial. *Of course* you can have just one. Who is in charge here, you or a bag of greasy snack food? Come on. Be a woman. Suck it up. You *can* have just one, or two, or as many as you want to have, but don't pass the buck. It's your mouth. It's your plate. It's your hand, moving the food from your plate to your mouth. If you want to do it, fine. Take ownership. If you don't, then quit whining and just don't.

Day Three Breakfast

Keeping in mind the concept of eating whatever you want but not all at once, let's start with your day three breakfast. You might want to eat the same thing you ate on Monday or Tuesday, and that's fine. You can always go back and review those chapters. But today, let's talk about one of the most popular breakfast foods, and how to make it work for you, if you like it. I'm talking about cereal.

For Cereal People

If you are one of the cereal people, good for you. Cereal can be a great investment, if you choose the right cereal. Oatmeal is a superstar, one of the nutritional choices, nutrient-dense, filling, and full of fiber. Oatmeal is also a great canvas for other flavors, like cinnamon, maple syrup, or vanilla extract. It's also perfect for colorful fruit like strawberries, blueberries, or cherries, fresh or dried. Plus, it's quick and easy to make at home. Regular rolled oats are good and natural steel-cut oats are even better.

You probably already know that packets of oatmeal sweetened with maple and brown sugar aren't the best investment, because they contain so much sugar and are processed. Oatmeal counts as a carb serving, and all that sugar in it counts as one of your sweets. However, these packets are small, so if you can eat one packet and be happy, I'm not going to argue with you. Ideally, you would choose the plain packet and add your own, more natural sweetener, such as fruit or honey. Personally, I need more volume in my oatmeal than I can get from one of those tiny packets, which seem like nothing to me.

BETHENNY BYTES

When I have to travel for business, I know I need a good breakfast to give me energy and stay with me for a while. Today, I went to Au Bon Pain at the airport and looked at all the bagels and huge muffins, and I knew those weren't going to be good investments for me. Instead, I chose a medium-sized oatmeal. I sprinkled a little cinnamon and brown sugar on it, and it was a fab choice. I ate half, then carried the rest onto the plane with me and ate that during the flight.

There are plenty of other hot cereals besides oatmeal. Try cream of wheat, hot barley cereal, or my Healthy Brown Rice Breakfast, at the end of this chapter.

If you like cold cereal, try to cultivate a love for the dark-colored, whole-grain, high-fiber cereals. The light-colored puffy cereals are full of sugar, have hardly any fiber, and don't fill you up. They aren't a good investment, because you'll be hungry in an hour, unless you keep filling up your bowl again and again, and that's not what we're doing. We're having one small bowl and enjoying it, remember? You don't have to measure or obsess. Just use your small bowl, put some cereal in it, and enjoy it with a little soymilk or low-fat milk (or whatever you really love and some fresh fruit).

I'm not going to give you a list of cereals. Just look at the back of the box. Make sure that you can pronounce all the ingredients, and that the cereal has some fiber. Don't be scared off by the few extra calories in a dense bran fiber cereal. This cereal will stay with you a lot longer. Add some fresh fruit, and don't refill the bowl again!

You can tweak your cereal experience to make it even better. If you love creamy milk on your cereal, have some, but if you don't care that much about the milk, use nonfat milk or low-fat soymilk. Or put some cereal in your yogurt instead. The protein in the milk will help you balance the carbs in the cereal, but the fat in the milk is necessary only if you really want it.

You can add a lot of things to cold cereal, to make it a better investment. Try a light sprinkle of dried cranberries, a few walnuts or sliced almonds, or some fresh in-season berries.

Also, be very choosy about your cereal. Look for cereals without added sugar and try for at least 5 grams of fiber in a serving. A little honey, agave syrup, or raw sugar on this kind of cereal is a much better investment than cereal presweetened with high-fructose corn syrup and processed white sugar. And yes, I admit, sometimes I put artificial sweetener on my cereal. Or just put some berries on it and forget the sugar. If you get used to sweetening your cereal with fruit only, sugary cereal can start to taste sickeningly sweet. Your palate can learn to prefer foods with less sweetener if you work on gradually training yourself to use less sugar. I used to put two and a half packets of Equal in my coffee. Now, when I have coffee, a dash of soymilk is plenty of sweetness for me.

NATURALLY THIN THOUGHT

Eating sweets makes you want more sweets. Avoiding sweets makes you want fewer sweets. Remember that before you make your decision. Just factor it in.

Day Three Lunch

Today, as you will be doing every day, balance your lunch on the basis of what you had for breakfast. If you had cereal with milk, then your body probably wants some protein and vegetables for lunch, rather than something full of carbs, but listen to your food voice to be sure. On cereal days, I like to have a salad for lunch, topped with some lean protein like chicken, fish, or some tuna salad with mayo and a little less dressing.

Today, I also want to talk about something that's taboo in a lot of "diets." What if (are you ready for this?) you actually *don't have time for lunch*? Don't faint; this is not a heretical statement. This happens to me a lot, and I'm guessing it happens to you. You aren't going to see any diet books telling you to skip lunch, but this isn't a diet; this is real life.

On some days, lunch is easy. You have a plan to meet friends, or you are at home and you make something good for yourself. But on other days, you might be traveling or in meetings or running back and forth from somewhere to somewhere else. Maybe you had a good, hearty breakfast such as oatmeal, yogurt, and walnuts. You aren't very hungry and your food voice isn't crying out for you to put on the brakes, so you just keep going until dinner.

OK, seriously, don't freak out. I am not telling you to skip lunch. If you are hungry today and it's time for lunch, have lunch. If you are the type of person who is likely to rip into the breadbasket like a wild animal if you skipped lunch, then you *must not skip lunch*. You have to ♡ *know thyself.* ♡ Remember, I am not telling you what to eat, or what not to eat. I just want to be frank about real life, and how sometimes, lunch doesn't work out. I know myself and I know when the time bomb is ticking and I have to eat. I also know when it's not a big deal. That's where you can be, too, but it never hurts to have an energy bar in your purse, for emergencies. My new favorite is the Greens brand, which is chocolate-covered.

So if you missed lunch, you missed lunch. It's not an excuse to go overboard at dinner. It's just something that happens sometimes. Don't make a big deal about it. I'm just telling you that if it works out that you don't get around to lunch on some days, that's perfectly normal, natural, and part of life, especially if you are really listening to your food voice, rather than to some idea about predetermined times when you are supposed to eat. Naturally thin people don't always get around to three squares a day. You don't have to, either, if you don't really feel like it.

BETHENNY BYTES

Guess what I had for lunch today. That's right, nothing! I was on a plane until 3 p.m. on my way to my class reunion, and had to deal with a business crisis. I hardly noticed because my good, solid breakfast of oatmeal carried me through and I was too busy to think about food. Will the dietary experts tell you to skip lunch? No way. And I'm not telling you to do it, either. I'm just telling you that you shouldn't eat if you don't feel like eating and you know you can skip a meal every now and then without losing total control later in the day. ♡ *Know thyself.* ♡

Day Three Dinner

Whether you had cereal, eggs, or a muffin for breakfast, and whether you had soup, salad, a burger, or nothing at all for lunch, at some point it will be time for dinner. Once again, what you have for dinner must depend, for the sake of balancing your account, on the meals and snacks you've had so far throughout the day.

If you did begin the day with cereal or another carb-laden food, and then you stuck with protein and veggies for lunch, you are probably ready for your second carb meal of the day. For many people, that means pasta. But people also have a strong and sometimes even fearful reaction to pasta, so today, let's talk about pasta and what it means for someone who is naturally thin.

Pasta

If you went through an Atkins/Zone/low-carb stage, you might still feel suspicious of and resentful toward pasta. It tastes so good, but it's so evil, right? Actually, that's not right. If you like pasta, you should eat pasta. Don't eat it every day of your life (that's not balanced), but enjoy it now and then. You can eat it smartly, making it into a good investment instead of a bad one. It's all in how you balance it.

One of the more important things to do when you eat pasta is to load it up with vegetables and have a salad or a bowl of soup first. If you fill yourself up on the vegetables and then eat just a little of the pasta, you'll be making a good investment. Don't make the mistake of filling up on the pasta and being too full for the vegetables.

Choose whole-grain pasta, if you like it and it's available. Cover it with vegetables and tomato sauce, or a tiny bit of whatever sauce you like. If you are eating white pasta, just be aware that refined flour spikes your blood sugar, especially if you eat a lot of it, so keep your portion very small. Just a cup of white pasta is plenty for you to really taste and enjoy the pasta experience without overdoing it. If you add lots of vegetables, one cup of pasta seems like three.

If you like olive oil and garlic on your pasta, as I do, fine, but realize this might be all the fat you need for the day. I also love linguine with clam sauce, but I eat the clams first, and just some of the linguine. Enjoy a few amazing bites, then stop. If you had cheese on your salad, don't put cheese on your pasta. You made your choice. But if you'd rather have a little high-flavor feta or Parmesan on your pasta, that's fine. Shave it on with a microplane (one of the tools from Chapter 5) so you get just enough to flavor the pasta without drowning it in fatty cheese. And leave the cheese off the salad. *You can have it all, just not all at once.*

BETHENNY BYTES

I'm out of town today and I missed lunch because of traveling. At 6 p.m. I had a SkinnyGirl Margarita, then I went off to happy hour with some friends. I certainly didn't eat any of the disgusting food that was offered. This is one of the nice things about paying closer attention to your food. When the food is bad, you won't wolf it down. You'll turn up your nose at it.

But by dinnertime, I was definitely ready for something more substantial. At the restaurant, I ordered a Greek meze platter. Meze is the eastern Mediterranean concept corresponding to appetizers, hors d'oeuvres, or tapas. It's small, tasty finger food, and in my opinion, it makes a great dinner. My meze platter contained hummus, roasted red peppers, falafel, and a bit of Greek salad. It was totally plant food but had enough protein and fat to be filling and satisfying. I also had a glass of wine. It was a great dinner, and fun to eat. (Remember always to include some protein in a meze or tapas experience like this one.)

You've put your pasta in a small bowl, right? Now you will be full on good investments, yet participating in a dish that you might have

HEAVY HABIT

Don't you just love Italian food? The pasta, the garlic bread, the wine, the tiramisu . . . Hold on a minute. That's not balanced, and real Italians don't eat that way. If you are going to eat pasta, skip the bread and the wine, or the bread and the dessert. That's way too much starch and sugar. Or, *taste everything, eat nothing,* having just a few bites of bread, a few bites of pasta, a few sips of wine. These foods all encourage you to eat more and more and more, so you must not overload on any of them, let alone all of them. If you are all about the dessert, then skip the wine, or just taste the tiramisu. Life is about choices, and you have to pick your battles. *You can have it all, just not all at once.*

thought would be forbidden forever on a "diet." Plus, that heavy, tired feeling you used to get after eating pasta will be a thing of the past. You'll feel great eating pasta in this way.

Now, I do need to clarify that when it comes to pasta, there are a few things I forbid myself, and I recommend that you avoid them, too. Fettuccine alfredo, macaroni and cheese, pesto-laden pasta drenched in oil, lasagna, stuffed shells, baked ziti, creamy vodka penne—all those really creamy-cheesy-oily pasta concoctions are so full of fat and calories that to me, they're not worth eating. I consider

BETHENNY BYTES

Sometimes I end up snacking a lot because I'm hungry. Sometimes I don't snack at all. It just depends on the day. Today was not a really hungry day. You might think I would have wanted snacks today because I didn't get a chance to eat lunch, but it's just not how the day worked out for me. You never know. Instead of eating because it's "time" to have a snack, I eat when I want to eat.

these to be "taste only" items. They are perfectly fine for a two-bite "exception." Remember, no food is forbidden, but many foods just aren't good investments, so it's smarter to eat them only in small amounts, and only when you really, really want them (never just because they are there).

However, if someone else orders something decadent like this in a restaurant, it's perfectly fine to try one or two bites. You don't have to be afraid of these foods, because you are now a person who can taste them, appreciate them, and walk away. But ♡ *know thyself.* ♡ If you can't yet control yourself around foods like this, avoid them for now. The day will come, and you are working toward that goal.

Here's a summary of what I ate this Wednesday, plus a summary of what I ate on two other Wednesdays. Remember, this is just to give you ideas. I'm not telling you what to eat.

Day 3 Recipes

Try these quick and unusually tasty recipes for a fresh take on cereal and a deliciously healthy linguini.

Healthy Brown Rice Breakfast

I've never understood why more people don't eat rice for breakfast. Brown rice is full of nutrients, fiber, and energy that stays with you for hours. Try this easy recipe the next time you have brown rice left over from the night before.

Serves 1

½ cup cooked brown rice

¼ cup soymilk (or use rice or almond milk, or regular milk if you like it)

1 tablespoon dried cranberries or raisins

1 teaspoon sliced almonds

1 tablespoon maple syrup

½ teaspoon cinnamon

Combine all the ingredients in a saucepan and heat over medium heat until warmed through, about five minutes.

Spinach, Chive, and Ricotta Linguini

I love this easy pasta recipe. It seems really elegant but only takes a few minutes. This recipe is for multiple servings, but fill up on a salad or soup first. Servings of pasta should be pretty small.

Serves 8

2 tablespoons toasted pine nuts

Salt and pepper, to taste

1 pound spinach or other linguini

2 tablespoons olive oil, divided

1 bag baby spinach, washed

2 cloves garlic, minced

1 cup ricotta cheese

½ cup freshly grated Parmesan, plus additional for finishing

2 tablespoons chopped chives

1. Toast the pine nuts briefly in a small nonstick skillet over medium-high heat, stirring constantly. Watch closely because they can burn quickly.

2. Bring a pot of salted water to boil and cook the pasta according to package directions.

3. Meanwhile, in a separate large nonstick pan over medium-high heat, heat half the olive oil, then add the spinach and garlic. Sauté until the spinach is wilted, then season with salt and pepper. Turn off the heat.

4. When the pasta is finished cooking, add it to the spinach mixture with a slotted spoon. Add one spoonful of pasta water. Stir in ricotta and Parmesan cheeses and toss well. Season with additional salt and pepper, if necessary.

5. Mount the pasta on a platter or individual plates and sprinkle evenly with pine nuts, chives, and additional Parmesan. Serve hot.

Chapter 15

DAY FOUR: THURSDAY

You're halfway through the week. How do you feel? Think about how your habits are changing, which things you find most difficult, and which things take hardly any effort, and survey the week so far as if you were looking at your bank account. (You've heard that before!)

Are you balanced? Are you in the driver's seat? Do you feel good about the way you've budgeted so far? Stay focused on *you*. It's better to take a close look at where you might have fallen down than to pretend a problem isn't happening. Knowledge is power. It's better to know you spent all your money than refuse to look at your bank account balance because you don't want to know the truth. It's the same with your diet. Be honest with yourself so you can be free.

Today, I also want you to think about rule 5: ♡ *downsize now!* ♡ Every time you eat something today, put it on a small plate or in a small bowl, and don't forget to make it beautiful. Take pride in the beauty of your food. Perfect small bites of delicious food arranged attractively on a sanely-sized plate will make you happy and satisfied. Are you ready?

Day Four Breakfast

Today is a new day. With every meal and every minute, you have another chance to make a smart decision that will help you feel and look better. So let's start the day right. Let's talk about those bread-y faves: bagels, muffins, English muffins, toast—some of the most popular breakfast foods.

If you are a bread-for-breakfast person, you might be thinking you can't possibly trade in your bagel, toast, or muffin for anything else. You *love* your bagel, toast, or muffin. I know. So here's my lecture for bread-for-breakfast people (like myself).

For Bread-for-Breakfast People

I will never tell you that you can't eat a bagel! Some people are very attached to their bagels, toast, English muffins, or whatever. If that's you, that's perfectly OK. No food is off-limits, remember?

But if you like bread for breakfast, you need to be smart about how you eat it. So let's think about this rationally. Remember that *you can have it all, just not all at once.* It's not what you eat. It's how you eat, and how much you eat.

Reality check: you know perfectly well that a giant muffin, even if it's "low-fat," isn't a good investment, especially when it's covered in sugar and nuts or frosting. Beware the humongous fat-free muffin, masquerading as a health food. You can't trust it! It's *not* calorie-free. The simple truth is just this: if it tastes soft, sugary, and delicious—if it tastes like cake and leaves oil on your fingers and the bag—then it's a muffin-shaped cake. You are eating cake for breakfast. Don't kid yourself.

I'm not saying you should beat yourself up about it, though. You can eat cake or a cookie or a slice of pizza or anything you really want to eat for breakfast. Just don't lie to yourself by thinking that you aren't really eating whatever it is.

But this doesn't mean that you don't want it, or even that you can't have it. If you really want a muffin (cake), get the best one—the lesser of evils—that looks good to you. Maybe it will be whole-grain or bran, or have fruit or nuts in it. Just be sure it's really worthwhile to you. Choose the one you want.

Then cut it in half, and don't you dare eat the other half!

I mean it. Those cakey muffins have a huge amount of fat and sugar. Give the rest to a friend or save it for tomorrow or just throw it away. It's too much food. Better in the trash than in your stomach. You paid to enjoy the muffin. This doesn't mean you have to enjoy every super-fattening bite. Taste it and move on. Don't worry that you aren't getting your money's worth. What's a waste of money is to plaster it all over your thighs.

That's not the end of it. You also have to think about what the muffin will do to you. It's all flour and sugar, and that means you'll be ravenous by lunchtime because your blood sugar will spike, then crash. If you do have a muffin, try to have some protein along with it, to help balance your blood sugar so you don't spike and crash. Have a few nuts or a soy or low-fat latte (the smallest size is probably all you need). Maybe that muffin wasn't the best use of your funds, but the point is that if you really want it, have it. Just be aware of what you are doing.

Think of it this way. You've just bought a pair of turquoise leopard shoes instead of a black cashmere sweater, which would have been a better investment. But since you wanted the turquoise leopard shoes, fine. You bought them when you ate half that muffin. You can buy the black cashmere sweater next time. Or buy nothing next time.

And what if you really, *really* want to eat the other half of the muffin? It's your day, your choice. If you do eat it, just know that you are done with sweets for the day. You had your fun; you loved every minute. Now balance the rest of the day on the basis of that muffin.

Choices have consequences, so make them with that in mind. *You can have it all, just not all at once.*

Now let's talk about bagels and English muffins. There can be perfectly reasonable breakfast choices, unless they are as big as your head with a slab of cream cheese an inch thick. Come on, you don't really think you aren't eating about 1,000 calories when you gulp down that giant hunk of white flour and fat, do you? Even a so-called "whole-grain" bagel usually contains a lot of white flour. You should recognize this when you order one. It's rarely going to be 100 percent whole grain.

NATURALLY THIN THOUGHT

Every time I eat a bagel or a sprouted grain English muffin (Food for Life brand is my favorite), I *scoop* it. That's my word for pulling out all that extra bread from the middle of my half bagel or English muffin. I don't need it, and you don't, either. Don't think this sounds obsessive. It's not; it's just sensible, and a perfectly reasonable way to enjoy a bagel while cutting out a lot of the calories. You won't even miss them. Toast the bagel and add just a bit of cream cheese (the protein helps balance the carbs), a bit of butter (this counts as a fat choice, so make sure it's worth it), a slice of low-fat cheese or soy cheese, or a very thin smear of peanut butter. My favorite way to eat a bagel or an English muffin is with a light smear of real butter and a slice of soy cheese. That's just my preference. Whatever you like, keep the portion small. Trust yourself. Don't lie to yourself about how much you are eating.

If you love bagels, you can be smart about those, too. A whole wheat bagel may not be the best bread choice in the world, but it's still a better choice than a white bagel or a sweet sugary bagel (blueberry, brown sugar, or whatever). So go ahead. Get the bagel. Eat half. Throw the other half away. You aren't depriving any starving children; you are saving yourself from junky calories you don't need.

As for the notion of "low-fat" or "reduced fat" bagels or cream cheese, let's talk about that for a minute. You know, we love to lie to ourselves. We see a two-cent printed sign or label that says "low-fat" or "reduced fat," and we think that gives us license to eat twice as much. I even catch myself thinking this sometimes, telling myself that the so-called "reduced fat" or "low-calorie" food is somehow a more virtuous choice and better for me. A lot of major companies have gotten into trouble for misrepresenting their products on the label. You can't trust advertising, but of course we all *want* to trust advertising if it tells us we can eat a lot of something. Trust yourself.

BETHENNY BYTES

Today, I left on a short trip with a friend and his kids. I woke up in the morning feeling thirsty, so I had a grapefruit at 9, with a bottle of Synergy Kombucha. Grapefruit is a great morning thirst quencher, and so low in calories that it's practically like eating air. An hour later, I was hungry. At 10, I had two scrambled eggs on half a scooped-out bagel with just a bit of butter. This was a good investment. It wasn't lunchtime yet, but my food voice said *eat,* so I did.

What I had was have a light fruit snack (mostly liquid) first thing in the morning, because I wasn't hungry yet. I waited until I was hungry to eat my breakfast because I don't wake up and shove food into my face just because the clock says it's time for breakfast. At least, I don't do that anymore. The point is that every person, and every day, is different. One day you might need something light early, and a later breakfast. The next day, you might be hungry first thing. Your food voice will tell you which day it is.

Speaking of weird breakfasts, a few weeks ago, I was on the *Today* show and the crew members, who had been working since their 2 a.m. call, were having lunch—BBQ, in fact—at 9 a.m. For them, it was lunchtime. Do what works for *you.*

Look, a bagel is made out of a bunch of flour. If you want it, scoop it, put something good on it, enjoy a few great bites, and move on with your life.

You can make even better choices for topping your bagel. What about a scrambled egg or a few scrambled egg whites on top? Great protein, and you probably won't even need butter. (But have some if you want it. Just a little.)

Day Four Lunch

Sometimes, you are going to eat lunch on the run. I know how it is. You get busy and you simply don't have time to sit down and have a well-balanced meal. That's reality. But it doesn't mean you have to eat junk. You can make smart choices whether you are in a convenience store, a deli, or a fast-food drive-through.

Obviously, you won't always make the perfect choice, or even a smart choice. When you don't, recognize that and balance it into your day. Make your next choices accordingly. Sometimes, it's a matter of choosing the least of a slew of evils, when you don't have time to sit down and eat a salad, a big bowl of vegetable soup, or something else you know would be a good investment. Sometimes I have time only to grab something really fast, and I choose a small bag of pretzels and a piece of cheese. The pretzels give me energy but not nearly the fat I would get from a bag of potato chips, and the protein in the cheese helps balance the carbs and keeps me satisfied until I can sit down to a more rational dinner.

Recently, I was on an airplane dying for something sweet and the only options were a massive Three Musketeers candy bar, a bag of mixed nuts and fruit, and a giant cookie. I thought for a moment, then wisely chose the candy bar and the nut mix. I ate half the candy bar and four almonds to balance all that sugar. This certainly wasn't an ideal lunch, but it was the best of the worst, it satisfied me, and I didn't run for food the second I hit my destination. Later, I had half a turkey burger and a big salad, to balance out all that sugar.

CELEBRITY SECRETS

I shot a segment for *People* with pop artist Brooke Hogan about what to eat on the road when she was on tour. She was often faced with nothing but Mini Marts and fast food and trying to eat something on her tour bus. I helped her figure out how to get the best of both worlds—junk food and smart food choices. Say you are at a fast-food restaurant. You might think a salad is the best choice, but if you have the creamy dressing with fried crunchies, nuts, croutons, sugary mandarin oranges, or bacon on it, it's actually more fattening than a small hamburger. If you really want a burger, get one. If you really want fries, get a small order, with the smallest burger and a garden salad. If you really want the milk shake, skip the burger and fries and get a small garden salad. Pick your battles and choose what sounds best—the *one* thing that sounds best.

When you have a sugar craving at the Mini Mart, go for hard crunchy cookies rather than the soft cookies that get oil all over your fingers. Look for protein bars with ingredients you recognize. And remember protein if you are eyeing candy. A Snickers bar is better than a pure chocolate bar because it has some protein. Also look for food with fewer ingredients. I like Charleston Chew because it has something like seven ingredients, instead of, say, twenty-five.

Some chips are better than others. Terra chips, soy chips, baked chips, or even Fritos, for example, have just a few ingredients, such as corn, oil, and salt. Others have huge lists of unpronounceable ingredients, and I avoid these like the plague. A lower number of ingredients often means a simpler, cleaner, more real food—even in a Mini Mart.

Obviously, this applies to any meal. Stuck in a mall or at an airport for lunch with only a food court? You might choose a small hot and sour soup and a small order of white rice, along with a side order of vegetables. That's a pretty good lunch, if not ideal, and it's making the best of what you've got. The point is that you won't always be perfect or even nutritionally sound at a given meal, but as long as the overall balance of your meals over the course of the day or even the week is smart and sensible and you never eat too much of any one thing, you'll be fine.

BETHENNY BYTES

Still on the road, we had planned to stop for lunch, but the kids fell asleep so we decided to skip it. Nobody was very hungry anyway. However, by afternoon, we were all hungry.

We stopped for a restroom break and I had a sweet tooth, so I browsed through the gas station shelves of junk food and picked out a Charleston Chew. This candy bar has fewer calories than a lot of other options, and I like it. It is chewy and takes a while to eat. I had two delicious bites, then gave the rest to the kids. I also got a bag of pretzels and had just a handful. Then I drank a lot of water. This was certainly not an ideal "lunch," or even lunch at all. It would have been a better investment if I had gotten some cheese or some other source of protein. But that was today. Sometimes, you aren't in a situation where you can make the best possible investment, so I did the best I could. I satisfied my snack-food cravings but didn't overindulge.

Day Four Snack

Some days, your snack and your lunch may morph into a single eating event. On other days, you won't want a snack. But if you do, remember to choose something smart. Here are a few ways to upgrade your snack choices:

- Instead of potato chips, choose pretzels or soy or baked chips if you want salt. Choose raw veggies with hummus or bean dip if you want crunch.
- Instead of nachos or pizza drenched in cheese, have a slice of cheese and a few whole-grain crackers. If you do choose a slice of pizza, choose one with vegetables on top, blot the oil and eat only half of the slice. Do you really want the whole crust?
- Instead of a large, fake, frozen yogurt ice cream with toppings, have low-fat ice cream or yogurt, or have one small scoop of

real, full-fat ice cream, and enjoy every bite. It's liberating! Preferably, choose a more natural brand like Ben & Jerry's or Häagen Daz, both of which come in individual cups. The regular versions of real ice creams are very high in fat, but at least they contain real ingredients. Remember to ♡ *get real.* ♡ Better to have a couple of bites of the real stuff than a giant bowl of fat-free sugar-free "ice cream." Or, do what I do and go for the happy medium—Ben & Jerry's low-fat ice cream, with great ingredients, or a cup of sorbet, or even a popsicle. Read the label!

- Even better: plain yogurt with a little honey or real maple syrup and a handful of nuts mixed in makes a delicious snack. If you really need chocolate, add a teaspoon of mini chocolate chips. This is a surprisingly satisfying snack, in my opinion.

Day Four Dinner

For a lot of people, dinner is the biggest and most interesting meal of the day, and throughout the week, I've covered some basic dinner concepts such as salad, bread, and pasta. I'm not the kind of person who thinks you always have to sit down for a big, perfect dinner with meat, potatoes, salad, and dessert. You know me better than that. I'm much more likely to suggest picking the one thing you want and going with that, or else just taking little tastes of all the different things and filling up on side orders of veggies.

But I know that a lot of people like to focus on an entrée, so to-day, let's talk about the entrée. For most people, it means something based on protein.

The Entrée

When you are cooking or ordering an entrée, obviously, you should have what you want, within reason. Personally, I try to avoid anything fried, creamy, or drenched in oil. Of course, there are always exceptions, but those exceptions (fried calamari, lasagna, etc.) are mostly for tasting, not eating. ♡ *Taste everything, eat nothing.* ♡

If you want to order a delicious entrée, I suggest sticking to the basics. This is what I do. Maybe you really want a perfect, tender little filet mignon or a New York strip steak. Maybe you love broiled chicken or grilled salmon. Here's the exciting part, and my newest rule for you. It's not one of the ten; it's a special, secret, subrule.

Don't eat boring food.

Sure, broiled chicken breast or salmon filet is on every diet you've ever seen. *Yawn.* What's the point? Don't eat a plain, skinless piece of dry chicken or an ultra-lean sliver of beef if that isn't your favorite cut of meat. Decide how you want to invest. Do you want salmon with béarnaise sauce on the side? Have it. Do you want chicken sauteed with buttery mushrooms? That sounds good. Personally, I love New York steak. However, I have never ordered or eaten a whole steak. I like a small taste of rich meat, but not a huge amount. By this point in my life, I can't even imagine eating a whole steak. There is such a thing as too much of a good thing.

A lot of restaurants serve meat with sauce, which can enliven a dish and make it more exciting. But you don't need to drown your food. A tablespoon of rich delicious sauce is plenty. Or jazz up your meat with mushrooms, peppers, and onions. You can pile lots of veggies on meat to make it more fun.

Also remember that your chicken might be dipped in flour and fried. Top that with a buttery marsala sauce, and wow—a healthful chicken just became super-high-fat. Pick your battles—have the chicken breaded, *or* with the marsala sauce. ♡ *You can have it all, just not all at once.* ♡ If it looks great, taste it and enjoy it. Just don't wolf down the whole thing. You don't need all that. You're naturally thin. It's all about portions.

I am not going to treat you like an infant and tell you how many ounces of each kind of entrée to eat. But I will tell you not ever to finish your whole portion, especially in a restaurant that gives you more food than one person should ever eat in a single meal. To savor

HEAVY HABIT

This one's for all you low-carb people. I love a few choice bites of steak, but I also know that too much red meat isn't good for anybody. It takes a long time to digest and weighs down. Give your body a rest: don't eat red meat more than twice a week, and never eat more than a piece the size of a small sponge in one meal. You don't need it, and after a while, you won't want it, either. Living on slabs of meat and cheese will start to seem disgusting once you've been eating to be naturally thin following the ten rules in this book. Sure, you can certainly go too far the other way and eat too many "carbs," as the low-carb people like to say, especially if you are eating refined starches such as white flour and white sugar. But eating pounds and pounds of meat every day is no way to be healthy or naturally thin. You might lose weight at first, but I bet you will gain it back. Stop dieting and stop eating so much meat! You'll feel much better.

and relish your meal, you don't need to eat a lot. Eat half and leave the rest. ♥ *Check yourself before you wreck yourself.* ♥

Now let's talk about how you *design your dinner*. Remember that today (and every day from now on) you are focusing on the size and arrangement of your plate. When you cook or order dinner and sit down to enjoy it, part of the pleasure of the meal is how it looks. Would you eat a pile of brown goo just because it tasted good? Don't just throw your food onto your plate and then throw it into your mouth. Arrange it. Make it colorful and attractive. Add beautiful vegetables and little drizzles of sauce. Put a bright, colorful salad or warm hearty soup on the side. (For more on side dishes, see Chapter 18.) Cut your protein into a small, perfect portion, whether it's grilled steak or grilled tofu.

Then, before you dig in, take a minute to appreciate the beauty, the aroma, and the whole experience of the meal. Remember to ♥ *pay attention,* ♥ savoring every bite. ♥ *Pay attention* ♥ not just to the taste. Continue to appreciate the meal with all your senses. That helps make dinner worth the time, the effort, and the calories.

BETHENNY BYTES

By the time dinner rolled around, I realized that my lunch, from the convenience store shelf, had set me up to want junk food. But I knew I needed to ♡ *check myself before I wreck myself,* ♡ so at the restaurant, I let the kids help me out. One gave me a bite of a mozzarella stick, another gave me a corner of a turkey and Swiss panini and the broth it came with for dipping, and another gave me a tiny piece of cheese. I had a nibble of a biscuit, but it didn't taste good, so I didn't eat any more. I also had a glass of chardonnay. I balanced out the mess with a small salad with chicken. I felt as if I had eaten lots of greasy bar food, but in reality, I had eaten only a bit. It was a ♡ *taste everything, eat nothing* ♡ meal, and it worked for me.

Day Four Snack

Now that your day is over, have you had enough, or are you still craving something more? Sometimes at night, I want something sweet or salty. Sometimes I don't. The trick is to stay on track with your expenditures and savings. Keep them in balance. If you've already had a few servings of sweets today, skip this snack. Have a big glass of water and go to bed, or have a bit of protein, like some yogurt or a piece of cheese.

But if you haven't had sweets today, a few bites of something sweet at the end of the day are perfectly reasonable. Just put your portion on a small plate and put the rest away so you aren't tempted to eat more than you should. And what if you know you can't control yourself around sugar in the evening? (You know who you are.) ♡ *Check yourself before you wreck yourself.* ♡ Don't even start.

The more you eat to be naturally thin, the more confident you will feel that you won't wreck yourself. A few nights ago, I was at a movie premiere and I had a small handful of dark chocolate nonpareils. Just three. Once, I would have eaten a whole box, but now, that didn't even cross my mind. It's a great feeling when you get really good at this naturally thin way of life.

BETHENNY BYTES

After dinner, I had four bites of the kids' chocolate sundaes. Later in the evening, I thought about how I didn't make the greatest choices today, but I still really wanted something sweet at night. (Can you say "PMS"?) I happened to have a piece of BethennyBakes vegan chocolate cake, but I didn't want to get started on the whole thing, so I had just one tiny bite of the frosting. That's all I needed. But I did vow to have a better eating day tomorrow! This was not the best, most perfect example of a smart day of eating, and I realize that. The point is that I'm obviously nowhere near a perfect eater all the time. But I'm a real person, just like you, and I've learned how to be naturally thin in the real world. In these situations, just try to minimize the damage.

Day 4 Recipes

I love steak, but I also appreciate chicken if it's prepared with plenty of flavorful ingredients. Try this recipe, which uses goat cheese and sun-dried tomatoes. It tastes great paired with the next recipe, for spicy broccoli.

Goat Cheese and Sun-Dried Tomato Chicken Breasts

This is a very savory entrée.

Serves 6 (Slicing the chicken can increase the portions you get out of this recipe.)

6 boneless chicken breast halves

½ cup goat cheese (chèvre)

1 teaspoon dried Italian herbs (a mixture, or use just oregano, basil, or thyme)

1 tablespoon minced fresh Italian parsley

Salt and pepper, to taste

4 tablespoons olive oil

4 cloves garlic, minced

½ cup finely chopped sun-dried tomatoes (get the kind packed in oil, but drain them first)

1 cup full-fat plain soymilk

1. Cut a slit down the side of each chicken breast, creating a pocket.

2. In a small bowl, combine the goat cheese, herbs, and parsley. Put a spoonful of goat cheese inside each chicken breast pocket, dividing the mixture evenly between the 6 chicken breasts. Season the chicken breasts on both sides with salt and pepper.

3. Put a sauté pan over medium-high heat. Put the olive oil in the pan and sauté the chicken breasts, facing up, until browned. Turn them over and brown the other side, then heat until fully cooked. Remove the chicken breasts and set aside.

4. Add the garlic, tomatoes, and soymilk to the pan. Season with salt and pepper. Scrape all the bits off the bottom of the pan. Bring to a boil and simmer 5 minutes. Spoon the sauce over the chicken.

Roasted Spicy Broccoli

Roasting brings out rich flavors from vegetables. This recipe makes a great side dish with chicken, or any other hearty entrée.

Serves 4

4 cups broccoli florets

1 small red bell pepper, chopped into 1-inch squares

2 tablespoons extra-virgin olive oil

1 garlic clove, minced

½ teaspoon red pepper flakes

Zest of ½ a lemon

Salt and pepper, to taste

Preheat the oven to 400°F. Spread the broccoli florets in a roasting pan and roast for 15 minutes. Remove from the oven and toss with the remaining ingredients, then roast an additional 15 to 20 minutes, or until tender.

Chapter 16

DAY FIVE: FRIDAY

TGIF, right? You might feel relieved that it's finally Friday, but don't think you suddenly have license to go back to your heavy habits, just because it's the weekend. The good news is that on the weekend, you can still have it all (just not all at once). Listen to me: *you are not going to deprive yourself. You are going to participate and have fun,* whatever plans the weekend has in store for you.

Weekends are a bit different from normal workdays, though. So while Friday may start out like a "regular" day (whatever that is for you), chances are it's going to end a little differently from most of your weeknights.

Weekday or weekend, you can be present. Be present every day of your life. The only difference between the weekday and the weekend is your schedule, but the way you choose to eat is part of your life—and that doesn't change.

So today, I'll talk you through Friday, and today's rule I'd like you to focus on is one of my favorites: ♡ *Taste everything, eat nothing.* ♡

Sometimes, when I state this rule, people don't quite get what I mean. They think I'm telling them they can never again eat a good-sized portion of anything. Other people get it right away, and it's as though a lightbulb goes off in their heads when they realize they can eat anything they want using this rule. You understand the rule now, so let's work with it today, ♡ *taste everything, eat nothing* ♡ is the rule to remember and live whenever you are eating in a restaurant, going to a party, going on a date—you know, all those "Friday night" things.

HEAVY HABIT

Do you ever fear going out? I used to be afraid to go to restaurants that I knew had only fattening food. I would even turn down fun events because I was so petrified by the thought of eating too much. What a waste! I want you to quit being afraid and start living. Participate in your life. Just remember to ♡ *taste everything, eat nothing,* ♡ and you'll have everything to gain and nothing to fear.

Day Five Breakfast

We've covered a lot of different kinds of breakfasts throughout the week, mostly consisting of typical breakfast foods. But that's hardly the extent of your breakfast options, so today, let's talk about alternative breakfasts.

For Alternative-Breakfast People

If you like to think outside the box for breakfast, that's great. Anything left over from dinner, whether it's what you cooked or what you brought home from a restaurant, can make a perfectly decent breakfast. Why not have chicken with vegetables, spaghetti, an enchilada, or a cup of soup? Just be sure it's what you really want, and remember that even if it's leftovers, you still have to balance what you eat for breakfast with your choices for the rest of the day.

I admit that I don't do this very often. Every now and then, I'll have a slice of pizza or half a sandwich for breakfast. But I know some people who love to eat leftovers, or prefer to make something for themselves that isn't a "typical" breakfast. That's fine—it's your breakfast. Eat what you want to eat. But again, balance it with the rest of the day.

Let's talk about another scenario. Maybe you just can't get very excited about breakfast. You've probably had it drilled into your head: "Breakfast is the most important meal of the day." I know—I've heard this a thousand times, too. I used to wake up every day and eat without assessing how I felt or even whether I was hungry. I was so obsessed with food that I just thought I had to eat breakfast. All the "diets" told me I had to eat breakfast.

Well, things have changed for me. Some days, I wake up and eat immediately because I'm hungry. Some days, I eat one of the breakfasts I've described for this week. There are even days when I go through the takeout containers from the night before to see what still looks good. Some days I just have fruit or a smoothie. (But this isn't always sensible until you've adopted your new, good strategies, because unless it's combined with protein, fruit alone will make you hungry in an hour.) Sometimes, I don't want to eat right away, and I wait until I'm hungry. Sometimes, I never get around to breakfast, because I'm too busy.

But let's say that today, you are hungry. And busy. If you are an on-the-go type like me, constantly running out the door, that's not ideal when it comes to breakfast. But maybe the conflict is mostly in your head. If it's at all possible, make time to eat something smart. On most days, you have two minutes, and that's all it takes, especially if you've thought ahead and have something quick in the freezer. It pays to be prepared.

If you think breakfast takes time, think about these options, which you should be able to access in just a few minutes:

- Small bowl of whole-grain cereal with soy or skim milk
- Small microwavable packet of plain oatmeal sprinkled with a few nuts, a little cinnamon, and 1 teaspoon of real maple syrup
- Scrambled egg white with salsa in a whole-grain tortilla or half a pita
- Half a sandwich (such as peanut butter on whole-grain bread)
- Scooped, toasted wheat bagel with 1 slice of soy cheese or 1 scrambled egg
- Hard-boiled egg or two (boil some eggs when you have time and keep them in the fridge) with 2 or 3 whole-grain crackers
- Small container of Greek nonfat yogurt with a sprinkle of almonds or walnuts and fresh fruit
- Small-portion bag of mixed nuts and dried fruit
- Healthy leftovers from last night's dinner
- Energy bar. I know—I complain about these, but they aren't all that bad. Pick the one you like that has the most pronounceable ingredients. I like the brand Greens, covered in chocolate.

Seriously, it takes just a few minutes to prepare and eat oatmeal or bran cereal with fruit or a scrambled egg and toast. Is that really so much time, when the alternative is to have a factory-made breakfast out of a package? An even worse alternative is ending up ravenous and eating way too much food later in the day.

BETHENNY BYTES

This morning, I woke up hungry, but I wasn't sure what I wanted. I waited until I figured it out. I wanted pretzels. So I had about 15 twisted honey-wheat pretzels, Synergy Kombucha, and a soy latte with just a little bit of hot cocoa mixed in. Not your classic breakfast, but it was just what I felt like eating. The milk added protein, the tea helped fill me up, and the pretzels provided that crunch I craved, so this was a pretty good investment considering my strange craving.

Day Five Lunch

Are you already thinking, "I know I'm going out tonight, so I'd better skip lunch"? Don't do that. I've said this before, but on Friday it's easy to forget, so I'm reminding you. If you already know what you are going to eat tonight, you can plan your lunch around that and what you had for breakfast. But you aren't going to binge tonight. You are going to be participating in a way that's fun and sensible. So if you are hungry and you want lunch, have lunch. Spoil your appetite all day long.

Then again, maybe you aren't hungry. Have a light lunch, or skip it if you really don't want anything. But listen to your body—not to the clock, not to your perception of what's going to happen later, not even to me. If you are hungry, eat some lunch that will balance your account as you go through the day. If you are hungry, don't you dare skip this meal, or you will lose control later tonight, and you know how that goes—the food, not you, will be driving.

You are your own designated driver when it comes to food, so stay firmly in the driver's seat and be smart about this. If it's one of those hungry days, then eat something. You can fill up perfectly well on a salad, a bowl of soup, or both—or on whatever else makes sense as a balancing meal for your day. Then you'll feel great until it's time for dinner, and then you'll be ready to make more smart choices.

BETHENNY BYTES

For lunch, I had made chicken salad with some leftover cooked chicken mixed with soy mayo, grated carrots, chopped tomato, Dijon mustard, and Spike seasoning, on one slice of Ezekiel sprouted-grain bread. I topped it with lettuce and a slice of soy cheese. By the way, Spike is an amazing seasoning. I can't live without it!

Day Five Snack

If you know you want to have dessert tonight, don't have a sweet snack. Have some vegetables or fruit with protein, or a small amount

---

NATURALLY THIN THOUGHT

Sometimes, you need to deny yourself just a little, not in a painful way but in a way that allows sense to override your inner whiny child. Let me give you an example.

Recently, I had an egg white omelet full of veggies and feta cheese for breakfast. For lunch, I had a medium-sized bowl of veggie chili. In the afternoon, I had a small brownie. On most days, that would be more than enough and I wouldn't be that hungry at dinner. But on this day, I was just starving.

At about 8 p.m., it still wasn't time for dinner. I would be eating late with friends. I had half a grapefruit to distract me, even though I was craving something salty and savory. A grapefruit takes a while to eat, but did it work? No! And I knew better, because fruit alone, without protein, can cause a sugar spike and make me hungrier than before.

But I knew I had already spent on the brownie and that caloric (although nutritious) veggie chili, so this is when I decided to (drumroll: what are you expecting?) *suck it up.*

In other words, the fact that you are craving something doesn't mean you always have license to indulge the craving. Sometimes, you need something. At other times, you really don't. I'd had enough that day and I needed to wait for dinner. Sometimes you have to distract yourself, and being naturally thin *isn't always just skating along.* Sometimes, it is difficult. *You can have it all, just not all at once.* I'm not going to lie to you and tell you that this will never be a personal discipline, because it is. But it's a discipline that is *worth it.*

---

of healthy carbs, such as a slice of sprouted-grain toast with a little butter and soy cheese or some nut butter. But don't feel that you have to snack at all. If you know you can last until dinner with no problem and still make a smart choice tonight, then don't worry about the snack. Remember, snacks are *not* required unless you are really hungry, but they can be very useful for spoiling your appetite if you know you will be tempted when you go out tonight.

BETHENNY BYTES

For a snack, I had four tangelos. But that didn't cut it, so I also had a 3-ounce low-fat, wheat-free, vegan banana oatmeal chip cookie. I was tired today and when you are tired, you tend to eat more. Sleep is essential! Don't let yourself get too sleep-deprived. Sleep is a smart investment.

Day Five Dinner

It's Friday night, and for me, that often means socializing with friends. It also means that my friends and I will probably go out for drinks. I'm a social person and I drink alcohol. I enjoy the taste of tequila, and, frankly, I enjoy the ritual of making and having drinks with friends. I'm not going to pretend that's not me. It might not be you, but if it is, I want you to see how I manage happy hour and going out for drinks with friends without letting alcohol derail my self-control.

Drinking Alcohol and Staying Naturally Thin

Honestly, I envy people who don't drink. They seem to glow with health and probably have fewer lines on their faces and no dark circles under their eyes. On the other hand, a lot of research shows that moderate drinking really is good for your heart. Not everyone agrees with the research, but I don't eat or drink because of research. You already know that. You don't, either. If you drink red wine, you drink it because you like it. What I eat and drink is based on what I want, and on what I enjoy, as long as I can keep everything in balance.

HEAVY HABIT

So you had a few drinks and you aren't hungry? Don't get all excited, thinking that you are going to be able to lose five pounds tonight by skipping dinner and just drinking. This is a detrimental *heavy habit*. Most of the time, drinking and skipping food will backfire. Every now and then, you might be able to skate by, not eat dinner, and wake up with a flat stomach (and a hangover) but you'll be starving all day. Most of the time, you will end up binging on too much food late at night and waking up feeling bloated and disgusted.

In other words, prepare. Even if It's getting late and you still haven't had dinner, a great choice is sushi, from a restaurant or even from a supermarket. Have some miso soup, a salad, and some sashimi. Or, if you don't like sashimi, snack on a few pieces of leftover chicken, smoked tofu, or small amounts of some other protein. You'll feel much better in the morning.

That's why I usually drink in moderation. I stick to my rule of two drinks, maximum, during an evening, with the occasional exception. I nurse my drinks, and I have very specific rules about what I will drink.

So in this section, I want to talk about drinking and being naturally thin. I've mentioned this briefly in Chapter 11, but I want to go into more detail now. These are my personal rules for drinking alcohol in moderation, so I can still enjoy it and participate in life, but not let it trip me up and make me overeat:

- Drink only clear liquor and add only real fruit and a tiny splash of a sweet mixer. I never drink anything that is almost all mixer. Such drinks have hundreds of calories, for no real benefit. Learn to appreciate the subtlety of a high-quality liquor untainted by a load of sugar, and sip it over ice. For me, the perfect example is a SkinnyGirl Margarita (see the recipe at the end of this chapter). If you really like margarita mix, add just a splash to your tequila, to get the flavor without all the calories.

- Always choose clear liquor over brown liquor: white tequila over gold, white rum over dark, vodka or gin over whiskey or Scotch. To me, white liquor is cleaner and has fewer aftereffects.

- Almost never have more than two drinks during one event (a party, going out with friends, etc.). There might be exceptions—some days I have more than two drinks—but let them be exceptions, not the way you do things most of the time. Most of the time, two is my limit, period.

- Drink a glass of water after every alcoholic drink. This is very important. Don't skip this rule!

- I don't make a habit of drinking wine. Sometimes I'll have a glass of wine or champagne if it's appropriate for the situation. However, wine is higher in sugar and, at least for me, has more aftereffects the next day. I consider a glass of wine one of my sweet choices for the day.

- If you are drinking alcohol with a meal, really limit starchy foods such as bread, pasta, and dessert during that meal. Don't have more than a few bites of these foods. Instead, focus on protein and vegetables. Protein in particular is very important to eat while you are drinking. Have a salad with roasted chicken or grilled salmon instead of a sandwich or pasta. If you have more than two drinks, make the lightest choice in your food. The night you have five drinks is not the night to order pasta!

- Avoid those big sugary-sweet bar drinks filled with sour mix, coconut cream, and other forms of sugar. I've mentioned this before, but I'm going to say it again because it is very important. Bar margaritas, piña coladas, and daiquiris contain hundreds of calories and no nutritional value. What a waste! Instead, make up your own drink, based on these rules.

What to Eat When You Are Drinking

What do you eat if you want to relax with your friends and have a cocktail or a glass of wine? You focus on protein and vegetables. The protein will balance the sugar in the alcohol, and that food will stay with you longer.

In my experience, no one thing makes you fat. Alcohol doesn't make you fat. It's a combination of drinking, eating too much, having bread, dessert, peanuts, and more drinks. If you are going to drink, you need to eat protein. But I'm not telling you to order a massive steak or a whole lobster. You have chosen to drink, and this means that you need to eat a light but nutrient-dense meal. Keep it light and clean. You need only a small piece of fish with sautéed vegetables or a pureed vegetable soup and salad, or a salad and a small appetizer. How about an artichoke, Parmesan, and avocado salad? That would be perfect—vegetables, fiber, a little protein and calcium, and healthy fat. Then you can feel good about toasting with your drink. Good choices: sushi; shrimp cocktail (I always substitute cocktail sauce, a great naturally thin choice, for drawn butter); a salad with chicken. Really limit the starchy foods.

When you've settled on what to order—a salad and a side, maybe, or an appetizer, or whatever looks really good—then remember to offer everyone else a bite, and leave some on your plate. Enjoy it, but when you aren't really enjoying it anymore, stop eating it.

Also remember that you are focusing today on ♡ *taste everything, eat nothing.* ♡ You still need to balance what you are eating and drinking, but if people you are with are ordering food that looks really great—especially starchy food—and you really want it, then participate. Taste it. Just don't *eat* it. That lets you stay in control without being self-sacrificing. People won't hate you, since you haven't passed up the nachos or the crème brûlée, refusing to take a single

NATURALLY THIN THOUGHT

Whenever I go out with friends for dinner and drinks, I assess how I feel before I eat or drink one single thing. First, I ask myself:

- Am I eating just because I'm in a restaurant?
- Am I eating because I'm hungry?
- What do I really want to eat?

The worst thing you can do when you are dining in a restaurant is to refuse to consider ordering the food you are actually craving. If you push that craving aside, it will pop up later in the form of overeating or worse. In this case, I decided to order something healthy yet satisfying and apply my rule *taste everything, eat nothing.*

On a recent evening out, I started with bresaola and arugula salad with shaved Parmesan, olive oil, and lemon. Bresaola is low-fat, thinly sliced, delicious, somewhat salty dried beef; and arugula is a bitter green, high in antioxidants. This salad satisfied my craving even though the meat was thinly sliced and it had just a little Parmesan.

I instantly offered three friends a taste, eliminating the possibility that I would overeat. Salads and appetizers are great choices because they come on smaller plates and they fill up the plate, giving you the impression that you've eaten a lot.

Then, as always, I ordered side dishes. Side dishes are a key to the Naturally Thin Program. They often include vegetables, and they fill you up on less food. When everyone else is diving into pasta and veal in cream sauce, I'm eating my salad and sautéed vegetables and filling up on much less. However, I had a taste of the cheesy pasta on the table. It's important to participate and not fear the food. Remember, nothing is forbidden.

bite. You'll all be having fun, but you'll still respect yourself in the morning.

What about dessert? If you are having cocktails, forget about ordering dessert. You've made your choice. But once again, when it comes to dessert, I want you to participate in life. If someone else orders dessert and it looks really good, or if you're on a date and you don't want to be a bore, have a taste, or even two tastes. ♡ *Taste everything, eat nothing.* ♡ I typically stay away from large amounts of dense cake, but I'll have a few bites with the whipped cream or icing. Taste what you want to taste. Just be sure it's really worth it, and don't go overboard.

When it comes to dessert, you also have to ♡ *know thyself.* ♡ Drinking alcohol can lower your inhibitions and make you less able to stop eating, even when your food voice is yelling at you to stop. Can you taste a dessert and appreciate it, or will tasting it set you off on a sugar binge? If you know you won't be able to control what happens next, then say no to the taste. You've made your choice. Next time, maybe you'll choose dessert over a glass of wine.

Another choice I sometimes make: if I have wine or a cocktail before or with dinner, I'll have just one. For my second drink, I'll order an after-dinner drink. However, remember that after-dinner drinks are loaded with sugar and alcohol, and drinking a lot of them is definitely not good for your body. After-dinner drinks are *dessert*. But as always, I believe in participating, and I enjoy the ritual and special feeling of a large snifter glass and the aura of relaxation after a meal.

BETHENNY BYTES

Tonight, I went out with friends and had one SkinnyGirl Margarita, a mixed green salad with ginger dressing, one spicy crab hand roll with no rice, and one spicy scallop hand roll with no rice. I had a handful of edamame, and 3 pieces of sushi with rice. I also had fun with my friends, an essential part of the eating-out experience. If I had said, "I'll just have a salad," I would not have been much fun as a friend or as a date, and I wouldn't have enjoyed myself as much. Remember to participate in your life!

So here's how I do it. I order my favorite after-dinner drink with a lot of ice. I sip it very slowly—this isn't difficult, because after-dinner drinks are strong and sweet. I never finish even half of it. The ice melts down, the glass is half full, and I feel as if I drank more than I really did, because I was drinking mostly melted ice. And if everybody is pressuring you about dessert, just say you're having an after-dinner drink for dessert, since that's exactly what you are doing. This way, you are participating. You are tasting. And you won't ever have to feel anxious about whether or not you should order Frangelico, your favorite liqueur, or whatever it is you love.

Day Five Snack

One risk of drinking alcohol is that you can come home starving. But you don't have to. If you have eaten well all day and made smart, balanced choices, you probably won't be starving. Still, I'm not saying you won't be hungry.

Drinking can suppress your self-control. I used to get home after drinking and want to eat everything in sight, especially if I had skipped dinner. That doesn't happen to me anymore, but occasionally, I do want a little food before I go to sleep. You can have a smart,

---

BETHENNY BYTES

After I got home tonight, I really felt I needed something sweet to finish off the night. I'd had only one drink tonight and one vegan cookie for a snack in the afternoon (plus fruit), so I decided it would be just fine to have 3 bites of leftover chocolate cake. It was just right, and after I ate it, I didn't feel compelled to keep eating. I had a glass of water and went to sleep. I knew I had eaten too many sugary foods today, but I wanted this snack, so *I decided* to have it. (I was the one in control.)

balanced evening snack, even if you've been drinking. But remember to ♡ *check yourself before you wreck yourself.* ♡ Are you really hungry, or will eating set you off on a binge? If you can handle it, make a smart choice. If you've avoided sweets all day and if you've limited your alcohol consumption, you can even have something sweet.

You made it through Friday! Congratulations. Are you feeling great, and in control of your life? Are your new thin thoughts stomping out your old heavy habits? If some of those heavy habits are still hanging around, don't worry. Change takes time, but you are on the right track. Just stick with me. And now you've got the whole weekend to look forward to. Let's keep going.

Day 5 Recipes

Going out? Having a party? Try these SkinnyGirl drinks, which gives you all the fun and flavor of traditional cocktails, with a fraction of the calories. But remember not to have more than two. These drinks are strong.

SkinnyGirl Margarita

I mentioned this drink when I was on *The Real Housewives of New York City,* and it became a topic of conversation on Bravo TV network's online message boards. It's also been the subject of one of the most common questions asked to Bravo. Around the world, bartenders have become familiar with it. I invented this recipe because I love the taste of tequila but I hate the calorie count of the big sugary margaritas you get in restaurants. I always ask bartenders to make this recipe, and it's never a problem. Sometimes I also make it at home, for friends. It couldn't be easier, and you'll save hundreds of calories without sacrificing flavor. In fact, I think this margarita is much better than the kind made with sour mix and sweetened bottled lime juice. I like to dip the rim of the glass in raw sugar.

Serves 1 (You can double, triple, or quadruple it if you are serving others.)

2 ounces white (clear) tequila (100 percent agave). Count 1, 2 while you pour; no need
for measuring.

Large splash of fresh lime juice, or 4 lime wedges

Tiny splash of orange or citrus liqueur

A splash of club soda to lighten it, optional

Combine all ingredients over a glass of ice or in a shaker and stir. If
using lime wedges, squeeze them into the glass. If you want to garnish
the rim with sugar, rub a lime wedge around the edge of the glass and
dip it before adding the drink. You can also make it in a blender. Fill
the glass to overflowing with ice, then add the ice and the other ingredients to the blender and blend until smooth.

SkinnyGirl Piña Colada

Normally, this drink is extremely high in fat and calories, but not this sensible
version, which I demonstrate how to make on one of my diet.com YouTube
videos. As you can see, my amounts are fairly nonspecific. Just use a splash;
I never measure.

Serves 4

4 shots clear rum, (about 8 ounces). Just count to eight; no need to measure.

Splash of light coconut milk (about ¼ can)

Splash of pineapple juice (no more than about ½ cup)

4 fresh pineapple wedges

Fill half the blender with ice. Add rum, then the coconut milk and
pineapple juice. Blend until smooth. Pour into four martini or margarita glasses and garnish each with a pineapple wedge.

Lychee Martini

I made this recipe during episode 4 of the first season of *The Real Housewives of New York City* on Bravo network. It was a big hit with my friends. I
think you'll like it.

Serves 1

1 shot premium vodka (about 2 ounces). Count 1, 2 while pouring.

1 ounce (count 1) lychee juice (you can also purchase 20-ounce cans of lychees in their own syrup at a grocery store and puree them, reserving 2 for garnish)

1 ounce (count 1) club soda (a great way to lighten any cocktail)

2 lychees, for garnish

Combine ice, vodka, and lychee juice in a cocktail shaker. Shake well and strain into a chilled martini glass, adding lychees for garnish. Option: Rub the rim of the glass with fresh ginger and dip in colored sugar.

SkinnyGirl Sangria

This fruity, fantastic recipe is great for a summer party, when fruit is at its peak and you have a lot of people to serve. Make It in a big punch bowl or a couple of pitchers.

8 peaches, pitted and sliced

4 white plums, pitted and sliced

1 pound green grapes, cut in half

3 bottles Prosecco (an Italian sparkling wine)

One 12-ounce can Fresca or diet lemon/lime soda

One 12-ounce can club soda

Combine all the ingredients, and chill for at least 1 hour. Serve over ice.

Chapter 17

DAY SIX: SATURDAY

Now that the weekend is in full swing, you may be feeling like rewarding yourself or celebrating, or you might be enjoying some downtime. However you spend your Saturday, it's probably a lot different from the way you spend your Monday or Wednesday. I said this on Friday but I'll say it again: this is no reason to derail yourself.

My schedule is usually a lot different on weekends. Sometimes I sleep late; sometimes I get up early to go somewhere. Sometimes I've been out late the night before. Every now and then, I even stay in all day (although I admit that this doesn't happen very often). More typically, I'm traveling somewhere, or spending a lot of time with friends.

Because no food is forbidden and I participate in whatever activities are part of my day, on weekdays or weekends, I never have to worry about food or get anxious about what I'll eat at a social event. You don't have to, either. Just keep following the ten rules, and you'll sail through the weekend without waking up on Monday morning unable to button your jeans.

You *should* be able to enjoy good food, the food you want to eat, on the weekend, but that's also true on any other day. You might eat out more often on weekends, but that's no reason for anxiety anymore.

Just don't use Saturday as an excuse to go crazy and forget all your rules. That's not the way to be naturally thin. Remember to ♡ *check yourself before you wreck yourself.* ♡ That's the rule I want you to focus on today.

Actually, I want you to focus on two rules today:

♡ Check yourself before you wreck yourself. ♡

♡ Cancel your membership in the Clean Plate Club. ♡

Both these rules are especially relevant on the weekend, when you might be more prone to overindulge, and when you are also more likely to be hanging out with friends, giving yourself lots of opportunities to get rid of some of the food on your plate, so you won't eat as much. If you all share, nobody gets as much, and that will help you to be naturally thin.

Also remember to leave some of your food. If I'm in a restaurant that serves huge portions, I often leave half my food, or take it home for later. I'm not unrealistic. I know that every now and then, you're going to polish off the whole thing, especially if it's something really good for you and you know you've made a good investment. But if you are ordering appetizers and sides instead of entrées, eating the "whole thing" is less of a big deal, so that's just one more reason to go in this direction.

One thing I almost always do—and this has become a part of my life—is to leave at least two bites, especially when I'm eating out. This is a great practice because all those two-bite pieces of food really add up over a week, a month, a year. I don't think twice about it anymore. I just leave some. Think of all the food you get to taste, but how much of it stays *off* your waistline because of those two bites (or more) you leave on your plate at every meal. It's a powerful rule and a tool for being naturally thin.

But back to Saturday. A lot of people like to go out to eat on weekends, and some of those people are all about going out for breakfast. So let's talk about that.

Day Six Breakfast

I often grab something from somewhere for breakfast, but I'm not one of those people who tend to go out for breakfast, sitting down and spending a lot of time in a restaurant. I'm more likely to get something at a deli.

But some people love to go out for breakfast, or find themselves out for breakfast fairly often just because that's how their lives are set up. If that's you, or even if you are like me and tend to order breakfast from a deli counter, let's talk about what you can order for breakfast, and how it differs from eating breakfast at home.

Going Out for Breakfast

In some towns, going out for breakfast is practically a religion. People like the camaraderie, they like the food, and it's just a part of their lives. If you are a fan of the big breakfast, I suggest you consider your breakfast *brunch*. You don't need to eat a big breakfast and a big lunch, unless you are physically very active. Balance. Let a big meal be two meals.

Now, let's think about breakfast in restaurants, and what that means. First of all, the fact that a restaurant can serve a four-egg omelette with four strips of bacon, four sausage links, potatoes, gravy, and four slices of toast doesn't mean you are compelled to order or eat all of that food. You will never have a good excuse to eat huge amounts of fattening food. It's simply never a good idea.

But this doesn't mean you can't eat some of all those things. You can look at breakfast as an experience in which you ♡ *taste every-thing, eat nothing* ♡; or you can focus more on the rule that ♡ *you can have it all, just not all at once.* ♡ Either way, you are going to ♡ *check yourself before you wreck yourself.* ♡

NATURALLY THIN THOUGHT

As the weekend wears on, busy or relaxed, are you remembering to be good to yourself? Get enough sleep. Move your body a little, in a way that's fun. And let yourself enjoy life, participate, and have fun. It's the weekend! It's not about food; it's about giving yourself a break.

But don't think this means your breakfast, or brunch, *can't* be a good investment, because it most definitely can. An egg-white omelette filled with vegetables and a slice of whole wheat toast is a very smart choice. You can even eat it all! But a sausage-and-cheese omelette? Need I say more? It just depends on what you want.

First let's consider eggs. I like eggs and I eat them for breakfast frequently when I wake up hungry. If you make eggs at home, you can take out some of the yolks (or not). You can use nonstick cooking spray instead of butter or oil. You can go heavy on the veggies and light on the cheese.

Ordering eggs in a restaurant is different. You have no idea what the people in the kitchen are doing, but if you are in a diner (read: greasy spoon), you can bet that butter and oil are involved. They are probably frying your eggs in a ton of grease, adding way more cheese than you would add at home, and not putting in the veggies you would choose.

But that doesn't mean you can't have eggs when you go out for breakfast. It does mean that you can special-order.

Now, in general, I don't admire people who are always holding up the waiter by explaining in great detail all the elements they simply can't eat and why they need their food cooked in a special way. It's obnoxious, and you know that everybody within earshot is wishing these people would get it over with. On the other hand, if you are eating in a restaurant and paying good money for the food, you should get what you want, right?

You can strike a happy medium here. Let me give you an example. If you like eggs Benedict, it's not that big a deal to ask for it to be served over whole-grain toast instead of a white English muffin. Maybe the restaurant can use turkey bacon, although Canadian bacon is actually a pretty smart choice, high in protein and low in fat compared with regular ham. You can ask for the hollandaise sauce on the side, or skip it altogether. These requests aren't inconvenient and they shouldn't take up any more time than ordering the normal way. Decide what you are willing to concede in order to have the eggs Benedict, then enjoy them.

Making requests in order to have the foods you really want can also make you feel that you've participated. You *can* have eggs Benedict, even though "dieters" might consider it forbidden. You just want it in your certain, special way. This is largely about attitude. The reason you are special-ordering is *not* that you can't have eggs Benedict the regular way even though you want to. In other words, the reason is *not* that you are deprived. No, that's not it at all. You are special-ordering because you are, admittedly, a bit of a food snob and you enjoy your food only if it's prepared exactly the way you want it and in a way you know will make you feel your very best. Remember, you don't need to finish it all, either. Yes, that's much better. Now you're eating to be naturally thin.

Breakfast in restaurants is often a matter of choices. "How do you want your eggs? White or wheat toast? What kind of meat?" So you have a ready-made opportunity to customize your breakfast in a way you know will make you feel best. Poached eggs aren't cooked in oil. Wheat toast is better than white (although it still contains a lot of white flour, so go easy). Do you really need bacon or sausage? OK, have one piece. If not, skip it. Some restaurants have turkey or veggie bacon, too.

So, you don't have to be a pain or annoying to get the breakfast you want when you eat out. Just order an egg and a slice of bacon on wheat toast and a glass of skim milk, or a veggie omelet (egg whites only if you like that) with just a bit of feta cheese. Or eat half of a regular omelette with a slice of bacon. Or, have a fruit salad with nuts, a bowl of oatmeal with just a touch of brown sugar and some blueberries, or something else along those lines. These are all great breakfasts, common on restaurant menus. So order up.

BETHENNY BYTES

Today I had Synergy Kombucha at 8 a.m. It's all I wanted. But around 9, I was hungry, so I went out and ordered an egg-white omelet with spinach, mushrooms, tomatoes, and a sprinkle of feta cheese. Some days, I need the comfort of toast. On other days, I don't. My food voice tells me which day is which.

Day Six Snack

Depending on how late you slept and what you had for breakfast, you may or may not feel like a snack. One problem with hanging around at home on weekends is that you can tend to eat just because you are *bored*. You aren't doing anything else in particular other than relaxing, so your mind wanders to food. Or you see an ad for food on television or your computer, and suddenly you are convinced that you *must have that food*. This can also happen if you see a billboard or walk past a restaurant with a picture of food in the window.

Don't be fooled by tempting advertisements. The human mind is very suggestible, and this is why advertising works. Who is going to control your waistline, you or a billboard? Come on, you know the answer. You are in control here, not some corporate ad exec. So turn away from the pictures of fattening food and be smart.

OK, you won't always make the smart choice. I don't, either. Sometimes, on a particularly hungry day, you will invest in a snack that you know isn't the very best choice for your nutritional needs. I tend to go for ice cream. When I do, I know I've had sugar and fat, and I balance them with the rest of my day. Remember that ♡ *your diet is a bank account.* ♡ As long as you remember this, indulging in a snack when you really want one will work out just fine. Most of the time, you'll choose wisely. When you don't, just balance your account.

BETHENNY BYTES

For lunch, I wasn't very hungry, but I had a sweet tooth so I had a small strawberry smoothie from Jamba Juice, and a handful of nuts. It was all I wanted at the moment, so it wasn't really lunch; it was a late snack. I ended up having lunch around 4 p.m. So what? Sometimes on a weekend, you end up eating snacks when you usually eat meals, and vice versa. That's fine, as long as you balance the day. Because I had a late breakfast, I had a snack for lunch. That was today. Whatever choice I make tomorrow might be completely different, but you can bet it will balance out with my other choices.

Day Six Lunch

For me, lunch on weekends is a crapshoot, especially when I sleep late and have a late breakfast or brunch. No problem. If you're hungry, have lunch. If you aren't hungry, have lunch later, as I often do. Or skip it, if you really are still satiated from breakfast. Remember, you don't eat according to the clock. You eat according to your food voice.

For example, last week I had a piece of pumpkin bread at 12:20 p.m. I knew I would be having lunch at about 1 p.m. The old me would have deprived myself of that pumpkin bread, even though I really wanted it. Now, I know that I can have it. I also know I will adjust my meal accordingly. Maybe I'll have a salad and skip the bread.

That's living in the moment, instead of always looking toward the future, obsessing about the next dreaded meal that keeps you from doing what you really want to do *now*.

BETHENNY BYTES

By 4 p.m., I was finally ready for lunch, so I had the inside of a shredded chicken taco. I didn't want or need the tortilla, so I didn't eat it. I also had black beans, which were a good source of protein, but I skipped the rice because beans are also starchy, so it was going to be either the beans or the rice, and I prefer the black beans. Black beans are a better investment than white rice.

The tortilla chips looked good, so I had just a few, with a small scoop of guacamole. I remember when I used to avoid guacamole like the plague because I knew it was high in fat. Not anymore. I love the taste of avocado, so I have a small scoop now, when I'm in the mood for it. It's a healthy fat and a smart investment because it helps keep me full longer. I could also have asked for a soft tortilla for my guacamole, if I didn't want the fried chips. Some days, I might do this, and eat more. Today, I wanted the chips, but I ate fewer of them. Choose what you want—are you going to *taste everything, eat nothing,* or are you going to choose something more substantial?

Day Six Dinner

On Saturday night, I'm usually eating out. Who am I kidding? I eat out on most nights. But on Saturday, people are more likely to go out to nicer restaurants, just because it's the weekend. I talk a lot about eating out and how to do it in a smart way—fill up on soup, salad, or both; order an appetizer instead of an entrée; share; taste small bites of decadent food if someone else orders it;

etc. Keep following all those rules. Most important, remember to *cancel your membership in the Clean Plate Club.* Don't eat the whole thing.

Eating in a restaurant with friends is really fun when everyone shares, and if you are the first to offer your delicious salad, soup, appetizers, or whatever to other people at your table, they will follow your lead. Sharing brings the whole table together and makes the dining experience more interesting and exciting. And you'll be focused on sharing and commenting on the different tastes more than on just gulping down whatever you ordered.

HEAVY HABIT

Do you ever feel threatened when someone wants to share your food? Do you resist sharing? This is a diet mentality. When you are desperate to get every bite of your food because you know you are allowed only half a cup of whatever it is, then you aren't going to want to share. Of course not—you are starving! Starving people don't share their food. So quit starving. Eat what you want, eat enough to satisfy you without stuffing yourself, and be magnanimous. Share your food, and participate in sharing if others offer you delectable bites of whatever they ordered. You'll realize that eating really can be a lot more fun than it was when you were always on a diet. And you'll end up feeling more satisfied on less because you aren't so desperate. You'll also be more fun.

Don't forget to take some food home. Be sure not to finish it all. If you don't want it, give it to someone else, or just leave it on your plate. If you have a dog, as I do, you can always bring home an actual doggie bag.

Also, remember the rules for drinking alcohol, if tonight involves some of that. Try to stick to two drinks, have a glass of water after each one, order clear liquor instead of brown liquor, and go easy on the sugary mixers. I don't drink alcohol every time I go out for a meal, but when I do, I follow those rules and order my SkinnyGirl Margarita instead of a huge sugary restaurant margarita.

NATURALLY THIN THOUGHT

If you go to a restaurant that has a frozen margarita machine and everyone else is ordering a margarita, you don't have to feel left out. You can adapt the SkinnyGirl Margarita slightly, like this: one shot of clear tequila on the rocks, with just a small hit from the frozen mix machine. Ask the bartender to do this for you, and if you get a funny look, so what? It's your drink, and you should have it the way you want it. Plus, you get the same taste for a tiny fraction of the sguar and calories, and you won't get a sugar spike and a subsequent urge to binge.

Day Six Snack

On Saturday night, sometimes dinner gets lost in the shuffle of socializing. I always tell you to eat when you drink, but in reality, there are times when it doesn't happen. Try not to do this—at least snack on something with protein if you are having a drink. But if you get home and you really haven't eaten anything substantial yet and you are starving, *do not binge*. This is a difficult situation to be in, but you can still be the master of your life.

Choose something with protein and put a small portion on a plate. Put the rest away. This happened to me recently. I went out and had a few drinks and a few pieces of Parmesan cheese to help slow down the absorption of the alcohol, but I never had a chance to actually have dinner. I got home starving at 2 a.m.

Now, the old me would have gone crazy and eaten everything I could find. Not anymore. I knew I hadn't done a good job of eating when I should have eaten, so I made myself a small bowl of spaghetti with meat sauce. This had the warm, comforting taste of pasta I craved and the protein I needed. I made only a little, and it really helped me feel better. I woke up the next day, I wasn't mad at myself, I let it go, and I moved on to better investments. That's why I'm naturally thin.

BETHENNY BYTES

For dinner, I went out to a restaurant with some friends. I had two small slices of barbecued brisket. It was fatty and really delicious, and I savored every bite. I also had a small salad of romaine lettuce, tomato, chopped turkey bacon, feta cheese, and creamy Caesar dressing. Then I had one bite of a friend's crispy chicken with the skin. This was a meal with a lot of really decadent food, but because I just had a little of everything, I wasn't stuffed and I didn't feel guilty. I was in control. I *tasted everything, ate nothing.*

If I would had eaten a huge amount of food, I would have felt terrible in the morning. It's a great, powerful feeling to finally get to the place where food doesn't rule you. *You* decide what to eat, and you never have to be afraid of food again.

The week is nearly over, and the weekend is nearly over, too. But we still need to talk about Sunday, so let's keep going! You are forming new strategies and changing your heavy habits every day, getting more and more control over your relationship with food. And if you aren't already losing weight (although I bet you are), you will be losing weight soon. Sometimes, it takes the body a week or two to realize what you are doing, but when you eat to be naturally thin, you become naturally thin. Stick with me, and it will happen. It's a marathon, not a sprint.

BETHENNY BYTES

After I got home tonight, I wanted something sweet. I had skipped both alcohol and dessert at dinner, and had that one scoop of ice cream around noon, so I knew I could afford one more sweet. I had half of a thin slice of Italian cheesecake I had left over in the refrigerator. Just right.

Day Six Recipes

When you really want brunch but you are cooking at home, consider these recipes. You can watch me prepare both on my diet.com YouTube videos.

Creamy Greek Yogurt Breakfast

This is a simple 1-minute breakfast using Greek yogurt, which is delightfully creamy but low in fat. This makes an amazing quick breakfast and also looks elegant layered in glasses for a breakfast parfait. Or have it for a satisfying snack.

Serves 1

¾ cup fat-free Greek yogurt
2 tablespoons blueberries
Sprinkle of raw sugar or sweetener
1 teaspoon slivered almonds
¼ cup Kashi Good Friends cereal (or your favorite cereal)

Mix everything together and savor every bite.

Faux Pancakes

I'm strongly against fake food, but I call this "faux" because it is actually an egg dish. This is a great protein-rich breakfast when you are craving something sweet. The small amount of sugar gives it just the right degree of crispiness. This is delicious and so easy. You can also make delicious French toast by dipping whole-grain bread into this mixture instead of making it into faux pancakes.

Serves 1

¼ cup liquid egg whites or two egg whites

1 whole egg

¼ teaspoon strawberry extract or vanilla extract

1 teaspoon raw sugar or sweetener

Fresh fruit or small bit of maple syrup or both

1. Heat a nonstick pan over medium-high heat. Spray with nonstick cooking spray.

2. In a bowl, mix egg whites, egg, extract, and sugar. Pour the egg mixture into the pan and stir lightly.

3. When the egg is firm on one side, carefully flip it over. When it is fully cooked and fluffy, carefully move it to a plate.

4. Top with fresh fruit or a bit of real maple syrup, or both.

Chapter 18

DAY SEVEN: SUNDAY

By today, I hope you are feeling different—not different in the sense of feeling like somebody else, but different in the sense of finally being able to start being *you*. Your food noise has quieted down, and your food voice is getting louder and clearer. You're feeling more and more like someone who is naturally thin.

But don't be frustrated if you still aren't feeling totally in control. It takes time to establish new patterns and break bad habits, but you are getting there, one day at a time. This is life. Every day is different. Every day, do the best you can, but don't beat yourself up when you make a choice you regret. Just keep going. With every choice, the scales shift slightly; and with every bite you take, you have an opportunity to balance that with all the bites, sips, snacks, and meals to come.

The longer you stick with balancing, the more you make ♡ *your diet is your bank account* ♡ a personal mantra, the easier this gets. I promise. It is worth a little effort to shed what's holding you back and weighing you down. You can be naturally thin, and you are already on your way.

Today, on the last day of the Naturally Thin Program, I want you to think about the rule 10: ♡ *Good for you.* ♡ You remember what this rule is about, right? On this day of rest, think about how you can design your life in a way that is ♡ *good for you.* ♡ A well-rounded approach to this goal will be to move your body every day, in a way that is kind and that you enjoy, even if it's just walking; to get enough sleep; to live your life and participate in the world; and to love yourself for exactly who you are right now. Without that, you won't be able to do this, because you won't really believe you deserve to be naturally thin. But you *do* deserve it. So let that be who you are.

Day Seven Breakfast

Yesterday, I talked about going out for breakfast. Today, the discussion is similar but not exactly the same. If you like to eat a big breakfast, then there is no reason why you can't combine the first two meals of your day into one spectacular meal. Brunch doesn't mean stuffing yourself. It just means that you want to eat a little more than you would at either meal—but less than you would eat in two complete meals. So actually, you end up saving. Brunch can be an excellent investment.

NATURALLY THIN THOUGHT

My latest craze is to eat a grapefruit in the morning during the winter, and watermelon in the morning during the summer. I tend to be thirsty all the time, and these juicy fruits really quench my thirst. An apple isn't this juicy, so it can leave you wishing you had chosen apple juice instead. But grapefruit or watermelon is just as good as juice, in my opinion. Eating juicy fruits is like having a long, thirst-quenching drink of pure juice—but with fiber.

You can have brunch in a restaurant, or maybe you like to make it at home. Either way, brunch doesn't mean huge portions. It can mean foods you wouldn't normally choose for breakfast, or breakfast foods along with more midday choices, or a glass of wine. Brunch is a great opportunity to apply the strategy *taste everything, eat nothing,* especially if you are having brunch at a breakfast buffet with a huge number of different offerings.

If you are faced with a breakfast buffet—at a restaurant, or of your own making—you do have to be careful. I've seen buffets where you would be overstuffed even if you just tasted everything. Do one lap around the buffet first to see what really looks best. If you see several things you want, select accordingly. Plan your plate in order to taste them all while still balancing.

And go up to the buffet only once!

But knowing you are going up only once is no excuse to heap your plate with a bunch of mediocre food you don't really want, just because it's there or because you paid whatever-ninety-five for the buffet. Be discerning. Naturally thin people don't bring back a mountain of food from the buffet, or if they do, they leave most of it. Watch them and you'll see. Make your choices. This is your chance

---

HEAVY HABIT

Some people worry that they really aren't getting their money's worth if they don't overindulge at a breakfast buffet. Do you ever find yourself shoving it in because you paid for an "all you can eat" meal? Let's deconstruct that argument. This country has increased its portions to absurd sizes. And more than half of Americans are now overweight or obese as a result. So people end up spending hundreds of dollars on diet programs, diet systems, diet foods, and diet books. So what's the most economical choice, really? Step back and see the big picture, and you'll understand that eating *less* at the breakfast buffet is the real steal.

to be a bit of a food snob. And if you've chosen wisely you may go back to get more good investments.

If it turns out that only one or two things look really good, or if you want to go to the custom omelet station and avoid the buffet altogether, then you can focus on rule 2— *You can have it all, just not all at the same time* —as a strategy. Quantity doesn't usually equal quality.

BETHENNY BYTES

Today, I went to Sunday brunch at noon, after waking up late. I had a delicious egg-white frittata made with spinach, mushrooms, onions, and tomatoes. The vegetables really made this a filling meal, but it had virtually no fat, so I knew I could indulge in something higher in fat later in the day.

Day Seven Lunch

You just had brunch. Are you really hungry again already? Are you sure you aren't just bored?

OK, maybe you didn't have brunch. You had a normal breakfast. Then have a normal lunch. If you did have brunch but you find your stomach rumbling mid-afternoon, have a light snack. You don't need another meal, unless you want to have your dinner early.

But that's fine, too. I'm the first one to say not to eat according to the clock. If you had brunch at noon and you are ready for dinner by 4, then have it. Or, if you already have dinner plans, consider how

---

BETHENNY BYTES

Since I had brunch today at the typical lunchtime, lunch was irrelevant. I was fine until mid-afternoon, when I was ready for a snack.

---

all that will balance out for the day. Choose your snack accordingly. You can do this. It's not rocket science.

Day Seven Snack

After a good brunch, unless you are having one of those days where you just aren't very hungry, you still probably won't hold out until dinner. That's fine. If you get hungry at mid-afternoon, have a healthy snack. Then you'll feel perfectly in-control when dinner rolls around.

BETHENNY BYTES

By about 3 p.m., I craved something sweet, so I chose a ramekin of soy ice cream. That wasn't quite enough, so I ate just the frosting off a Bethenny-Bakes cupcake. Perfect! I didn't need the cupcake part, so instead of worrying about "wasting" it, I threw it away. This is naturally thin thinking at work.

Day Seven Dinner

After a weekend of eating out, you are probably ready to have a nice Sunday dinner at home. If you had brunch and haven't eaten since then, you are probably ready for a good-investment dinner. If you are the cook, then you can decide what kind of meal will balance your day. If you are cooking for your family, you can help balance everybody else's day, too.

Sunday is a great day to cook because people tend to have a little more time to devote to preparation. Some days, I'll putter around the kitchen all afternoon to prepare a good Sunday dinner. I don't do that every Sunday, but I do it when I get the chance because I love to cook. Maybe you don't, and that's fine. But if you are cooking at home, keep in mind the things we've talked about all week, including the different parts of a typical dinner: soup and salad, bread, pasta, entrée.

There is one more aspect of dinner we haven't covered in much detail, so let's talk about that today: side dishes.

Side Dishes

As I've mentioned, side dishes are one of the great skinny secrets of a meal. Take advantage of them. A side dish can even become the meal's centerpiece. When you cook at home, you are probably preparing a main course. That's fine. Make it, and have a small portion. But you will probably want some side dishes to go with it. To me, the side dishes are the exciting part.

Loving Vegetables

Side dishes are where vegetables really get to shine. I always like to include a salad with dinner because it's good to fill up on voluminous, fiber-rich raw vegetables. Side dishes add even more vegetable variety to your meal. I know that a lot of typical side dishes are based on starch—pasta, rice, bread. But if you want to be naturally thin, those aren't the side dishes to focus your efforts on, and certainly

NATURALLY THIN THOUGHT

The bulk of your diet should consist of high-volume vegetables, with a little fruit, some whole grains, and some protein. Eat vegetables every chance you get, whenever you feel the urge. The more you eat them, the more you will learn to appreciate them and even to crave them.

not the ones to fill your plate with. Instead, focus on beautiful, delicious, filling, nutritious vegetables.

Part of learning to love vegetables is making them spectacular. Roasted sliced Brussels sprouts will make your family feel as if they are eating potato chips because of the crispy leaves. Roast zucchini, corn, and tomatoes with basil and seasonings. This recipe knocked Gina Gershon's socks off when I cooked it on the set of Denis Leary's show. (See recipe at the end of this chapter.)

As for kids, teach them to eat and love vegetables *now*, and change their lives for the better. I say bring on the vegetables!

NATURALLY THIN THOUGHT

It's not exactly a side dish, but soup makes a great starter to a meal If you can get your family to eat soup as a starter, they will be filling up on something really good for them, not on higher-fat food. A good soup filled with vegetables is a painless, comforting way to add more veggies to your life.

Vegetables are best when they are in season, so pay attention to what is freshest and most local in your market. Go to farmers' markets if you have access to them, and you'll be getting vegetables that haven't been shipped across the country to get to you. They taste better and tend to have fewer chemicals on them. I usually buy organic vegetables when I have the option. I feel that they're better for me, and for the environment. Local vegetables are more eco-friendly, too, because they required a lot less fuel to get to you from the farm. Keeping all this in mind will help you to feel more connected to your food, and that makes dinner a lot more satisfying, in my opinion.

Easy on the Carbs

What about starches? You know whether you have eaten cereal for breakfast or pasta for lunch, and whether or not you feel like having a glass of wine with dinner. Now is when you decide whether your day has balanced out in such a way that you can have some starch with dinner. But remember that starches are very high in carbohydrates, and the more refined they are (white rice is more refined than brown rice, and white flour more than whole-grain flour), the hungrier they tend to make you feel after you've already eaten. Approach starchy foods with caution.

There are better starch choices and worse starch choices. In general, choose whole grain over the refined grain (like the aforementioned brown rice over white rice) and whole food over processed food (such as half a sweet potato or half a baked white potato over mashed potato flakes, white pasta, or macaroni and cheese from a box). Yes, sometimes vegetables are starch: this is true of potatoes, corn, and winter squashes like acorn and butternut. They all count when you are balancing your starch investments for the day. Be sensible and meet me halfway. By now, you know exactly what you need to do to change your life.

BETHENNY BYTES

For dinner tonight, I went to a Chinese restaurant with some friends. I had a half order of sautéed chicken and vegetables. It was oily, but I'd had barely any fat today, so that was just fine and in perfect balance. I also had three large sautéed shrimp with scallions and ginger. In Chinese restaurants, choose the lighter-colored sauces if you can. They tend to be lower in fat.

Day Seven Dessert

And speaking of carbs, if you feel that you must have dessert with dinner, look a little more closely at this feeling. Are you just in the habit of dessert, or are you really craving something sweet?

I like to wait for a while after dinner before I decide whether I really want dessert. Sometimes it takes a while for you to feel really full from dinner. You have to stop eating for a few minutes and pay attention to your food voice. If it turns out that you really do want dessert, keep the dessert small: a few sips of liqueur, two bites of a decadent dessert, or a small bowl of something a little more restrained, such as low-fat ice cream, frozen yogurt, or fruit. That should be enough to give you a feeling of participation and of self-indulgence, without losing control of your daily balance.

BETHENNY BYTES

In the evening, at about 9, I had a sweet tooth, so I ate five small pieces of licorice. It was chewy and sweet and just what I needed to feel satisfied for the day.

Now that Sunday is over, don't look ahead to Monday with such dread that you feel you need to bury your feelings in food late at night. Instead, look at Monday (and every day) as a new opportunity for eating well and making smart choices. Take a bath to relax and go to bed early if you need to catch up on your sleep. Remember how important sleep is to your health and your appetite control!

And don't worry about the occasional slipup. You're fine, and you're doing a great job. Just keep going. One meal at a time.

Day Seven Recipes

These are two of my favorite recipes. I love roasting vegetables, to bring out their flavor. And who doesn't love brownies, especially when they are low in fat but taste sufficiently decadent to feel like a weekend indulgence.

Pan-Roasted Zucchini, Corn, and Tomatoes

When I made this recipe on the set of Denis Leary's show, *Rescue Me,* Gina Gershon tried it and was crazy about it. I bet you'll like it, too. This is great to make in the summer when zucchini, corn, and tomatoes are all at their best.

Serves 2 to 4

1 teaspoon olive oil

2 medium zucchini, cut into 1-inch pieces

1 clove garlic, minced

Salt and pepper, to taste

Corn cut from 1 ear

½ cup pear tomatoes, cut in half (These are like cherry tomatoes, but pear-shaped. If you can't find them, grape or cherry tomatoes will also work.)

1 tablespoon fresh shredded basil leaves

1. Heat a nonstick skillet over medium-high heat and coat lightly with the olive oil. Add the zucchini and garlic and season with salt and pepper. Stir constantly so garlic doesn't burn, until the garlic is lightly golden brown.

2. Add corn and tomatoes, and cook until the zucchini is tender. Add the basil just before serving.

Amazingly Moist Low-Fat Brownies

You would never know these delicious brownies are low in fat.

Serves 8

1 cup raw sugar

6 tablespoons unsweetened cocoa powder

1 cup plus 2 tablespoons part skim ricotta cheese

6 tablespoons egg whites

⅛ teaspoon salt

1 teaspoon vanilla extract

½ cup plus 1 tablespoon oat flour

1 teaspoon vegetable oil

Cooking spray

Preheat the oven to 350°F. Combine all the ingredients in a bowl, then pour into a small brownie pan sprayed with cooking spray. Bake 35 to 45 minutes, rotating the pan halfway through, or until a toothpick inserted in the middle comes out clean (check after 30 minutes).

Chapter 19

GOING FORWARD

The week is over, and now that you've spent seven days with me, working through the Naturally Thin Program, Monday is rolling around again.

People like to say they will start their diets on a Monday. I say there is no Monday. There is only this present moment. You might have started a diet before, and fallen off it. That's frustrating, but that's not you anymore. Now you are starting your *life* again, in a fresh new way that will help you grow and change beyond your wildest dreams. The time is now, Monday or no Monday, whatever day it is. Don't wait. Right now is the only reality.

But you also need to look at your life in context. You've worked with me for a week, or maybe more, if you spent time reading the first ten chapters of this book before you began the Naturally Thin Program. That's fine, but now that you are at the end of the book, you might still feel as though you are on shaky ground.

This is completely natural. You've spent a lifetime acquiring heavy habits and you can't expect them to evaporate in just a few days or even a few weeks. If you still feel you need a lot of practice with the rules and strategies, turn back to day one of the Naturally Thin Program and let me guide you through the next week. And the next, if you need it. I'll be here for as long as you need me.

I like to read things more than once, and I believe that reading these chapters over again a few times will help plant the seeds of new, healthy, naturally thin thinking firmly in your mind, so those seeds can grow and become part of your life. But if you want to go solo this week, that's great, too! Just keep me close by for whenever you need advice, inspiration, or a well-meaning but firm nudge in the right direction.

Memorize the ten rules. Live them. And *live*. You've emerged out of fear and frustration and into a new way of seeing food, your life, and even the whole world. It's a new day, every single day, so be there for your life. You'll enjoy it even more, now that you know how to be naturally thin.

Appendix

Three Weeks of Bethenny Bytes

Here's what I ate over a period of three weeks, dutifully recorded just for you! Sometimes I met my goals and sometimes I didn't. Sometimes I had 3 protein meals, or 3 sweets, or not enough protein, or too many carb meals. But most of the time, I balance my accounts just about right, and that's the most important part. Remember, *this isn't a meal plan for you.* It's just here to show you how one naturally thin person eats, and to give you inspiration as you decide how you— as a fellow naturally thin person—will balance your own account each day.

WEEK ONE	Monday	Tuesday	Wednesday
Breakfast	⅔ of a spinach, mushroom, feta, and egg-white omelet; ½ whole-grain toasted pita (protein meal)	Watermelon and small cup of creamy hot chocolate (sweet)	Medium-sized bowl o oatmeal with cinnam and a little brown sug (carb meal)
Lunch	Big bowl of Japanese soup with vegetables, chicken, and soba noodles; a handful of edamame; and a salad. (carb meal)	Medium-sized bowl of chicken noodle soup with large pieces of white-meat chicken and a small number of noodles; half a tofu salad sandwich (protein meal)	None
Snack	Small bowl of low-fat Ben & Jerry's fudge brownie ice cream. (sweet snack)	Bag of Glenny's Multigrain Soy Crisps (savory snack)	None
Dinner	Large garden salad with cucumbers, tomatoes, marinated Italian vegetables, and small amount of feta cheese; ½ turkey burger; ½ a baked potato (carb/protein combo)	1 SkinnyGirl Margarita; small green salad with vinaigrette and added veggies; small cheese plate with olives and marinated vegetables (no bread); a few bites of New York strip steak; sautéed mushrooms; broccoli rabe. (sweet, protein meal)	Greek meze platter w hummus, roasted rec peppers, falafel, and Greek salad (carb/protein combo)

rsday	Friday	Saturday	Sunday
ergy Kombucha An hour later, crambled eggs on half ooped out bagel with a tiny bit of butter tein meal)	15 twisted honey-wheat pretzels; Synergy Kombucha tea; and a soy latte with a little hot cocoa mixed in (carb meal)	Synergy Kombucha tea (early); egg-white omelet with spinach, mushrooms, tomatoes, and a sprinkle of feta cheese (later in the morning) (protein meal)	Synergy Kombucha tea; egg-white frittata with spinach, mushroom, onion, and tomato; small slice multi-grain bread (protein meal)
harleston Chew dy bar; handful of zels b meal—and not a good one!)	Chicken salad made with soy mayo, grated carrots, chopped tomato, Dijon mustard, and Spike seasoning, on one slice of Ezekiel sprouted-grain bread topped with lettuce and a slice of soy cheese (protein meal)	Inside of a shredded chicken taco (no tortilla); black beans; a few tortilla chips; one small scoop of guacamole. (protein meal)	None
sed it	Four small tangelos; one 3-ounce low-fat, wheat-free, vegan banana oatmeal chip cookie (sweet snack)	Small strawberry smoothie and a handful of nuts (sweet and savory snack)	Small cup of soy ice cream and the icing off the top of a Bethenny-Bakes cupcake (sweet snack)
te of a mozzarella k; a corner of a ey and Swiss Panini the broth it came for dipping; tiny e of cheese; side d with chicken; glass hardonnay tein meal, sweet)	One SkinnyGirl Margarita; mixed green salad with ginger dressing; 1 spicy crab hand roll with no rice; 1 spicy scallop hand roll with no rice (protein meal, sweet)	2 small slices of barbequed brisket; small salad with Romaine lettuce, tomato, chopped turkey bacon, feta cheese, and creamy Caesar dressing; one bite of crispy chicken with skin (protein meal)	½ order sautéed chicken and vegetables, 3 large sautéed shrimp with scallions and ginger (protein meal)

(*continued*)

WEEK ONE (*cont.*)	Monday	Tuesday	Wednesday
Snack	Small bowl of Stonyfield Farms crème caramel frozen yogurt (sweet snack)	(At a cocktail party.) One deviled egg; a few sips of champagne (savory snack, plus one exception)	None
WEEK TWO			
Breakfast	Synergy Kombucha tea; ½ turkey with cheddar sandwich on whole-grain bread (go figure—it was in the fridge) (protein meal)	1 whole grapefruit; Synergy Kombucha tea; a little later: medium decaf soy latte (sweet)	Synergy Kombucha te (not really a meal)
Lunch	None	Small bowl of split pea soup; salad with turkey, tomato, feta, broccoli, carrots, and a light vinaigrette (protein meal)	Nicoise salad with a small can of tuna in water over greens, topped with olives, a teaspoon of capers, 2 boiled new potatoe cut in half, green bea tomatoes, a drizzle o olive oil, and freshly squeezed lemon juice (protein meal)
Snack	Hot pretzel from a pretzel stand (savory snack)	(At a publicity event) 1 piece shrimp tempura sushi, handful of edamame, 1 SkinnyGirl Margarita (savory snack, sweet)	Small rice bowl full o leftover linguine in an oily marinara sauce (savory snack)

rsday	Friday	Saturday	Sunday
g bites of kids' colate sundaes. er at night, one tiny of icing off a vegan colate cake eet snack)	3 bites of leftover chocolate cake (exception)	½ thin slice of Italian cheesecake (sweet snack)	5 small pieces of licorice (sweet snack)
le; medium decaf latte; slice of legrain toast with a e of soy cheese tein/carb combo)	Small bowl of leftover chicken lo mein (protein meal)	1 grapefruit, Kombucha tea (not really a meal)	Healthy tuna melt (scooped sprouted-grain English muffin, tuna, soy cheese); small salad with Romaine, turkey bacon, tomato, feta cheese, and creamy dressing (protein/carb tomato)
ad: Mesclun mix tomatoes, green ns, shredded beets, rinkle of crumbled cheese, a few k peas for protein, clear vinaigrette. croutons! ½ turkey ger with cheese but un; ¼ crabcake tein meal)	Tuna salad on toasted whole wheat bread topped with a slice of soy cheese, a slice of tomato, and sprouts (protein/carb combo)	Shared a salad of chicken, avocado, greens, and tomato; 5 or 6 rings of sautéed breaded calamari; ⅓ piece of whole-grain bread with a drizzle of olive oil (protein meal)	None
all low-fat vanilla ge ice cream eet snack)	Small handful of mixed nuts (savory snack)	2 BethennyBakes chocolate low-fat muffins (I really wanted 2 this time, although I usually have just 1) (2 sweets)	None

(*continued*)

WEEK TWO (*cont.*)	Monday	Tuesday	Wednesday
Dinner	⅓ of a Cobb salad with bacon, avocado, bleu cheese (I didn't eat the croutons or eggs); 3 shrimp with cocktail sauce; ½ baked potato; a few pieces of watermelon (protein meal, sweet)	A few sautéed mussels; a good spoonful of rich mushroom and meat Bolognese sauce with just a little linguine (the sauce was what I really wanted); sautéed spinach; 1 glass of chardonnay (protein meal, sweet)	1 SkinnyGirl Margarit shaved artichoke/ Parmesan salad, ligh dressed; a tiny bite of a friend's mozzarella; appetizer portion of grilled calamari over spelt (a grain); roaste tomatoes; 2 bites of a friend's steak (sweet, protein meal)
Snack	Small bowl of microwave popcorn (savory snack)	2 sips of Frangelico and a biscotti (sweet snack)	1 large bite molten chocolate cake; 3 sip: Frangelico on the roc (sweet snack)
WEEK THREE			
Breakfast	½ cup iced coffee with Silk vanilla soy creamer; ½ egg white omelet with feta, spinach, mushrooms (protein meal)	Synergy Kombucha drink (not really a meal)	Synergy Kombucha drink; grapefruit (not really a meal)
Lunch	Miso soup; 1 glass Chardonnay; 2 large prawns; arugula salad; side of sautéed mushrooms (sweet, protein meal)	Sprouted-grain English muffin with light spread of butter, one slice turkey bacon, and soy cheese (protein/carb combo)	Small arugula salad w grilled calamari (protein meal)
Snack	None	Small handful of nuts (savory snack)	Sprouted-grain Englis muffin with a slight spread of butter and a slice of soy cheese (savory snack)

rsday	Friday	Saturday	Sunday
ice of pizza, cut into hs so it seemed like slices; 1 SkinnyGirl garita (b meal, sweet)	1 glass of wine; small salad; small crabcake; just the cheese and sauce off a soggy piece of pizza (the crust was not worth eating) (sweet, carb meal)	½ Caesar salad (shared, no croutons), one bite each of: Kobe hot dog, short ribs, ravioli, steak (off a friend's tasting menu); crab cake appetizer (protein meal)	Glass of chardonnay, small portion of brisket, ½ order of rich and decadent mushroom risotto (sweet, protein/carb combo meal)
ne	None	¾ scoop coconut sorbet (sweet snack)	None
ergy Kombucha tea; decaf latte; 1 whole pefruit together, this is a b meal, even though ch element is so low-)	Hummus and roasted red peppers on one pita triangle (carb meal)	Scooped sprouted-grain English muffin with light spread of butter and a slice of soy cheese; Synergy Kombucha tea (carb meal)	Two bites of a cheese and spinach omelet; small order of black bean soup; glass of Chardonnay (protein meal, sweet)
ieces shrimp and cado brown rice hi roll otein meal)	1 glass Chardonnay; ½ spinach salad with crabmeat and hearts of palm (sweet, protein meal)	Small bowl of split pea soup; ½ salad with seafood and greens (protein meal)	½ of a tofu salad sandwich (protein/carb combo)
ll-scooped toasted eat bagel with a slice soy cheese and a tiny ead of butter vory snack)	Half a bag of popcorn with sea salt; one bite of a cookie (savory snack, plus an exception)	½ low-fat brownie (sweet snack)	Small cup of frozen yogurt (sweet snack)

(continued)

WEEK THREE (*cont.*)	Monday	Tuesday	Wednesday
Dinner	Medium Greek salad with feta cheese and chicken; 1 SkinnyGirl Margarita; a few chips with a small scoop of guacamole; roasted vegetable side dish (protein meal, sweet)	Small bowl of whole wheat pasta with grated pecorino cheese and a tiny bit of butter; 2 SkinnyGirl Margaritas (at a cocktail event) (carb meal, 2 sweets)	One SkinnyGirl Margarita; green sala drizzled with ginger dressing; 1 spicy scal hand roll with mayo but no rice; 2 steamed vegetable dumplings; 1 steamed crab dumpling; 2 pieces of sushi (sweet, protein meal)
Snack	Small handful of blueberry granola and almonds (sweet snack)	Slice of bread with black bean dip and one slice of soy cheese (savory snack)	Two bites of a friend's Pinkberry frozen yogu with sprinkles (sweet snack)

rsday	Friday	Saturday	Sunday
vl of spinach egg- te soup; small salad; nall pieces of chicken :ata)tein meal)	3 spicy crab hand rolls with mayo but no rice; side order of mixed vegetables; salad; handful of edamame (protein meal)	2 SkinnyGirl Margaritas; 3 pieces of Parmesan cheese; large salad (2 sweets, protein meal)	Cup of gazpacho; small serving of eggplant ratatouille; grilled fennel; glass of Chardonnay (carb meal, sweet)
all scoop of real ice am veet snack)	Four good bites of banana pudding (sweet snack)	Small bowl of spaghetti with marinara and a little bit of meat sauce (savory snack)	4 thin, crispy ginger cookies and just a couple sips of Frangelico (sweet snack)

Acknowledgments

As I sit down to consider all the people who have helped to launch me on the trajectory to where I am now, I feel humbled and grateful. I can't begin to name everyone and every experience that has helped bring me to this place, but I want to mention a few people who have made a big difference in my life.

First of all, I'm grateful to David Shanholtz aka "keebler" for helping me when my cookie business needed a boost. He had faith in me and helped me in ways that I could not have helped myself. Who would have imagined that something so small as buying a cheap video camera to film me selling cookies at a trade show would have led me to the *Martha Stewart: Apprentice* opportunity?

I would like to thank the Natural Gourmet Cooking School for giving me confidence and knowledge about food, its healing properties, and about the many wonders of health and how much it affects every aspect of our lives.

Thank you to Kevin Mazur, for believing that I could build a business, send a message, and that people would receive it. Thank you for helping to teach me this crazy business and to realize to "don't hate the player, hate the game." You shoved me down photographers' throats when they wanted no part of me, pushing me on red carpets to get my name out there.

Larry Butler, you are a lifelong friend. You have been a family member. You have always believed in me and told me that if I were a stock, you'd invest everything you own. That has always stuck with me. You have been my biggest cheerleader and rooted for me from day one.

Thank you to my mother for telling me at four years old that I was different and that there was a star over my head. Thank you John Parisella for treating me as your own.

Jill and Bobby Zarin, you have changed my life forever and you are the family I never had.

Keith Berkowitz, thank you for giving me the gift of Jeremy. Jeremy, thank you for believing in me, for being a great teammate and totally "getting it." Zach, thanks for taking the leap. Thanks to the great team at Touchstone Fireside. Lori and Joce, thanks for being on team "B" without ever wavering. Jake, thanks for Lori and thanks for pushing for me.

Thank you Keira and Jen O'Connell. You pushed me through and I will never forget.

Thank you to Bravo for welcoming me into your family. You gave me the space to be myself, be honest, and to let me shine. You are innovative and edgy and took a huge chance on me. Andy, Frances, Lauren, Cameron, and Christian—you really let me run.

Eve, thank you for having my voice, for living this book, and for making it your life. You are busy yet you threw your heart, soul, and family into this. You understand me and "get it" completely. This is the beginning of an infinite road together.

Molly, you are my touchstone, the oil that makes the wheels move. You are authentic and real and you came to me when the rocket launched and you helped me hold on.

Jason, thank you for your heart, for your soul, and for knowing that integrity is what you do when no one is looking. Thank you for pushing me to finish the book, for always putting yourself on the line for me, for encouraging me to never look back, and for putting yourself in endless situations, just to help me shine.

Last, Cookie, thank you for unconditional love, snuggling, and for your big furry heart.

I am so grateful to all of you. I know now that dreams do come true. If you want it, then go get it. Go big or go home!

Index